The Pilot Light Effect

by Maria Skelly

Cover artwork by Penelope Ball.

Edited by Simone Blais.

ISBN: 978-0-2285-0554-9

10 9 8 7 6 5 4 3

Printed in Victoria, BC, Canada

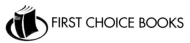 FIRST CHOICE BOOKS

www.firstchoicebooks.ca

This book is dedicated to:

My dear husband Kim, you are my strength and love, now and always. Together we are unstoppable.

To Harley Preston, personal trainer extraordinaire: Without you there would be no story to tell. You have instilled in me that my past does not define my future. You patiently continue to tackle my challenges with enthusiasm and determination. You have changed my world beyond measure.

You both make my world shine, and I thank you from the bottom of my heart.

Standing Strong

Life isn't always that fairytale dream
It can go so completely wrong
You find yourself tired and weary
This can't be where you belong

We deserve to be happy and healthy
Is that too much to ask?
And yet we find ourselves broken
Simply hiding behind the mask

Don't let what's in the past own you
It comes at too high a cost
Don't let each new day be
Something else for you to have lost

Take back your life
Stand tall and be strong
Be brave and believe
It's never too late to truly achieve

Table of Contents

Introduction

It's not until I look at things in hindsight that I realize how there were times that I was barely holding on by a thread. I can clearly see how on occasion, I inadvertently made things much harder on myself.

My life has been quite eventful. My Mum would always say to me, "Maria, challenges are character building." She was right, but how much character does any one person need? Sometimes it has been just a matter of coping, as best as I can. Physical challenges since birth, a serious car accident as a teenager, a sudden career change in my forties, and the worst of all, an unexplained medical decline that left me in constant mind-numbing neurological pain for more than a decade.

I muddled along, and had anyone asked me how I was doing, I would have said that I thought that I was coping reasonably well under the circumstances. I believed it, too, most of the time. I would keep myself occupied as best that I could during the day. It was when I was alone with my thoughts in the middle of the night that the reality of my situation would terrorize me. I got good at looking as though I had everything under control though. Fake it until you make it as the saying goes.

A friend of mine believes that people should come with an

instruction manual, and I think he might be onto something. Without any booklets or manuals, we have to make things up as we go. When it was beyond my capacity to understand the complexities of my situation as it was regarding my medical downturn, I relied on the professionals.

I got as many educated opinions of what I should do to regain my health as I could. It is only with hindsight, though, that I could see the error of my ways. I accepted what was unacceptable, and I didn't take steps to rectify my situation until it was nearly too late. I was in over my head, and had no idea which way I should turn.

When I heard doctors tell me, "There is nothing more we can do for you," there were only two choices that I could make: believe them, accept that nothing can be done and give into the darkness; or light a fire to guide my own way out.

It took every ounce of effort I could muster, but I found it: a small internal spark flickering away, my personal pilot light That light is my strength when I fear I have none, and the flame to propel me forward. When I started to give it fuel, it grew into an inferno you could see from outer space.

That was the fire that allowed me to tell the medical experts, "Thanks for all of your help, but I'll take it from here."

Ready to light it up? Let's go.

Part One

a few flickers

The First Sparks

The first time that I was ever consciously aware of the existence of my inner pilot light was when I was eight years old, and my parents decided to emigrate from England to Canada.

Eight-year-olds don't get to decide much, other than perhaps what toys to play with and clothes to wear. It would be at least another decade before I could really start to plan out my own future, so there was nothing I could do about my parents' plan. Canada here I come.

We emigrated a week before Christmas, and my major concern was whether or not Father Christmas would find me thousands of miles away from home in time to still deliver my highly anticipated gifts on Christmas morning. As an eight-year-old, these were the things that mattered.

I wasn't feeling particularly festive that year. There wasn't the customary thrill of counting down how many more sleeps until Father Christmas came. All I could think about was how many more days there were until we were due to leave. The few things we were taking with us to Canada had been packed. The house was down to bare essentials. There wasn't a Christmas ornament in sight.

I couldn't take all of my toys, so I had to choose just one or two of my most precious things that I could take with me on the airplane. I agonized over my choices and hated leaving some of my very favourite things behind. I was attached to my toys, and I worried about what was going to happen to them once I left.

It wasn't just the toys; I was leaving friends and family behind and these were the people I loved and felt safe with. I was going to have to find all new friends. I wondered what Canadians were like?

In school, we had learned about the British Isles and possibly a small part of Europe in Social Studies. If other continents were mentioned, I couldn't remember. My world knew nothing about North America and Canada, other than that my Dad had an uncle John who lived there.

Whenever Uncle John visited, he would tell my parents about how nice it was in Canada. I blamed him for planting the seed that made my parents uproot us all. Sure, I heard Dad say that it was for the good of the family, but as an eight-year-old I didn't know what that meant. Dad pointed out to me on a map where we were going to be living. It only confirmed how far away from home I was going. I could feel his excitement; but for me, Canada might as well have been another planet. We were going to stay with Uncle John until we got settled. Dad already had a job to go to. This was going to happen whether I liked it or not.

Even though I was filled with anxiety about my future, it was my pilot light that kept instilling in me that I could handle the move, although I was much too young to know it at the time.

The day of departure came. My aunt and uncle took us to the

airport and I bravely said goodbye to them and boarded the plane. I learned in that moment that I could be courageous, and even though I wanted to run. I could go into the darkness and survive.

I couldn't believe how long the flight took. It was my first time flying and it was eventful but boring. There were no movies to watch to pass the time back then. I had some colouring books and pencils, and Golly my soft doll if I wanted something to hug. That was it for my entertainment.

We should have had a quick stopover in Amsterdam; however, plans changed when the plane that we were going to fly to Canada on, had cracked its windscreen when it landed. I thought it was a sign that we shouldn't be going, but no one else would agree with me. We were all a little fed up by this point. The repair caused a delay of over 13 hours. This firmly convinced me that there was no hope now of Father Christmas finding me in time for Christmas. What would happen to my wish list? Imagine my alarm when I discovered that Father Christmas was going by the alias of someone called Santa Claus here in Canada. If my wish list was addressed to Father Christmas, would this Santa person even read it? Oh my gosh what if Santa wasn't the real thing? That's it, I am going back.

Gerard, one of my much older brothers had flown over about a month before us. Much to my relief, he had made certain that there was a Christmas tree up when we arrived. We were all exhausted by the time we eventually landed, and it took a few days to settle in. I was raring to go on Christmas morning, and yes, Father Christmas did find me. I remember

The Pilot Light Effect

running around in my pajamas telling everyone that he had found us after all. This was blatantly obvious, but somehow, it wasn't official in my mind until I had personally told each of them. I was truly astonished by the efficiency of the North Pole. The best part was that I got to replenish my toy supply.

Things felt normal while we were at home, because the whole family was there together. It was when we ventured outside that I was jolted back to reality that this wasn't England. I think one of the things that hit me as most peculiar was that although Canadians spoke perfect English, ordinary things were called something completely different, or sounded familiar and were spelled wrong. A tyre became a tire, the bonnet of the car was a hood, while the boot had become a trunk. Windscreens were called windshields and a lorry was a truck. Travel across the Atlantic and a lorry becomes Laurie, changing from a vehicle to a girl's name. My biro became a pen and the frock I wore was now a dress. There were some socially awkward things to avoid, too. In England, if you said someone's house was homely it meant cozy and nice. Say that to a Canadian and they would be most offended because you have just called their home ugly.

After the Christmas holidays my sister and I were registered at the local school. It would be the first time that I was in a public school and found it unsettling that the class size was much bigger and there were no uniforms. It was a lot to take in. The education system starts at age 4 in England whereas it is 6 in Canada. That put me clearly ahead of my classmates. Instead of blending in, I stood out, I spoke with an accent and had my hand up often to answer questions. This didn't make me popular; I came off as an unintentional know-it-all. These were questions I knew the answer to because I had already studied the subjects two years before. When no one else would answer the teacher's questions my hand would automatically go up.

So here I was, in a foreign country, with no friends and beyond bored. My sister was busy doing her own thing, and my brothers were at an age that they would be married and gone within the next couple of years. That gave me lots of time to think. I didn't make any friends that school year. I was all I had.

First lesson I learned was to like myself. As humans, we don't always do that. My theory even at eight years old was that if I don't like myself then that wasn't exactly a ringing endorsement when trying to convince other people to like me. I was my own cheerleader. That was the first building block to creating my inner spark.

I didn't go over the top and believe that I was suddenly the best thing since sliced bread. I reasoned that it was perfectly fine that not everyone would love me. No one gets that, not even celebrities, there would be people that didn't like me and that wasn't something to blame myself for. I liked some people more than others for no specific reason, and I was normal, so other people must be the same. As long as I liked myself, I would always have at least one friend. Whatever is out of my control, I let go of.

This is a helpful trait, letting go whenever possible, stops me from holding onto things, or as I call it, emotional hoarding.

It just creates way too much baggage for my liking.

The next thing I focused on was buckling down and doing the work. I wasn't finding that school year particularly enjoyable, and rather than shouting from the rooftops that I wasn't happy, I focused on the academics. I had the answers to get a good grade, so I turned my attention to get the best grades that I could and move on.

I have found in adulthood, that bad situations don't last forever. They just feel like they are lasting forever. So rather than using up my energy complaining about things I can't control, I focus on the smaller things, some detail I can do well. Because I became engrossed in that one thing, everything else just falls away.

This might seem a lot for any eight-year-old to comprehend and take on. I don't think that I knew that was what I was doing at the time. When you are building a fire and look at that first chunk of wood or the pile of kindling, it doesn't look like much on its own but put it all together and you have light and heat.

I did come to love being in Canada, but it all took time. I think about the cousins that now only know me from the few words I put into a Christmas card each year. I think about the family weddings we didn't get to go to, all the births we celebrated from afar. That one choice my parents made all those years ago irreversibly changed the course of my life. Not in a bad way, I've had a good life, it just instilled in me that other people can change your life, so you better always be ready for change coming from any direction.

Memories of a Lost Girl

I was always an awkward child. I never noticed the signs that I ran and walked differently than other children. My Mum and Dad would tell me that no one is good at everything, and as long as I was running and playing around having fun, it didn't matter. I had incredibly bad balance right from my earliest memories. If I was on flat ground, I managed reasonably well, but give me an uneven surface or rocks to climb, it was game over. When I walked along the beach I always tried to go to the flattest ones. If I came across larger logs, I would either try and go around them (which wasn't always practical), or I would sit and swing my legs over the other side, then get up and carry on. It didn't take much to stop me in my tracks if the log was too big, or if my feet couldn't touch the ground on the other side. Even if I was with other people I would just turn around and make my way back to where I started, my walk was done.

It's funny how people adapt. From a very young age, I began to make excuses why I didn't want to go for a walk or didn't like the beach if I knew that the walk would be too difficult for me. As a young child, it was okay, possibly even sweet, that I would hold onto Mum or Dad's hand for support, but by the age of 9 or 10 at the very latest, independence kicks in and holding your parent's hand is no longer cool. Even though I was insecure about walking alone, the need for independence, and protecting my image, won hands down. If I was with a close friend and needed help navigating something uneven, I would ask for their help on occasion, but it was only as a last resort. Once I had met my boyfriend Kim at 15, it was much easier. We held hands all the time and still do almost half a century later. I could always do more whenever he was around. He created the possibility of adventure and made me feel safe.

I had absolutely no natural ability for anything physical, and I still don't. My lack of agility would frustrate my gym teachers, and they would end up punishing me. I would get told in angry tones to go and sit in the corner so they could get on with teaching the other children, the ones who actually wanted to learn. I was wasting their time. I wanted to learn, and couldn't understand why they didn't see that. In fact, it has only been recently that I realized that none of it was my fault at all. It was because they didn't know how to teach me.

I grew up in a time when it was acceptable to hit children in school. If you didn't behave, you would be sent to the headmistress' office and given the dreaded strap. Thankfully that never happened to me. It was however a looming threat. One wrong move and the headmistress would be there ready with the strap waiting for me. If she was coming, we all knew it wasn't going to stop at one strike.

Although I successfully managed to avoid the strap, I was unable to escape punishment from my physical education teachers. I remember one hitting me hard across the back of my legs with a ruler whenever I tried to keep my balance walking along a balance beam. The strike would startle me so that I fell off of the beam. The teacher knew that would happen, and she hit me anyway. This would lead to fits of laughter among my classmates. That taunting laughter rang in my ears and remained with me long after gym class had ended. I always sarcastically thought, "Sure, go ahead and hit me. I'll learn better that way."

I would be able to walk a balance beam at the same time I would walk on the moon. Instead of exploring why I couldn't do something, I was treated as though my inability was an act of defiance. Would that make the choice to hit me socially acceptable? I dreaded going to gym class, it would keep me awake at night with worrying. This wasn't an isolated incident, either. As soon as balance practice began, out came the wooden ruler again. I knew what was coming. I would try and will myself to balance properly but the attempts were futile.

It didn't matter what sport I learned, I was hopeless. I couldn't get a volleyball to go over the net. I couldn't shoot hoops to save my life. Baseball was downright dangerous. I couldn't ride a bike and I didn't swim. Even when bowling, my balls lived in the gutter. I hated sports and my classmates resented me playing with them.

When it came to fitness, I was either a problem or invisible. Once, my gym teacher sent us out for a run. She ran with our class for the first few minutes and then, when we got to the start of the trail, she told us she would meet us at the other end. I think she wanted an easy class where she didn't have to do anything with a bunch of 15-year-olds.

I was going as fast as I could, but the trail was really uneven, steep and difficult. It wasn't long before I had lagged behind the rest of my class and found myself alone, lost, in the woods. I kept going along, running, breathlessly trying to catch up. I never did.

I was stopped in my tracks when I came across a fast-running stream. I hadn't a clue where I was at that point. My guess is that we were supposed to go through the stream and continue on, up the other side of the bank onto the road, and eventually back to school. Maybe I had taken a wrong turn somewhere and didn't know it. Surely we weren't supposed to have to cross a stream?

I made several attempts to cross that stream, none successful. I slipped trying to get across, hurt my ankle, and now found myself crying, wet, and frightened. My classmates were long gone, and there wasn't a soul in sight. It was a harrowing experience.

I was over 2 hours late that day finding my way back to school and I was a physical and emotional wreck. I was covered in mud from head to toe with all sorts of cuts and bruises. I was shivering cold, wet, hobbling as I walked, and just wanted to go home. Fortunately, it was pretty close to the end of the school day. I didn't even try to go to my last class. I simply sat on the curb and waited for my ride home.

I had expected to encounter some sort of fanfare upon my arrival. The search party was bound to be excited to see that I made it back in one piece. But no one had even noticed that I was missing. It was obvious by their actions that the faculty didn't care. I could have been laying on the trail seriously injured or dead. Why wasn't my gym teacher sounding the alarm? When I got back to school, I was asking if anyone had seen her and was told that she was teaching a class. She had abandoned me. She continued on with her day without a single thought of me. In fact, not one person asked if I was alright even though you only had to look at me to know that something had happened. My gym teacher should have counted heads as everyone got back from the run. Did she somehow lose count? What about the teacher for my next class? Surely he should have known that I wasn't there, and reported it to someone. I wasn't the type of girl to miss class. After years of feeling invisible in gym class, had I actually achieved invisibility? I believe so.

There was no one out looking for me, and my family had no idea of the danger I had been in. This was long before the days of mobile telephones and texting.

The only thing that got me through that day, was not letting myself give up. I didn't sit down and wait to be found. I did say a prayer or two, but I kept going, even when I didn't know where I was. I did my best to calm my heart down, take a deep breath, and look for signs of a proper path. I listened to that inner spark and it once again looked after me.

When I got home that night, I told my parents what had happened. They were alarmed and angry, rightfully so. This was a side of them that I had never seen before. Their outrage was not directed at me, their only concern was that I was alright. The next school day, Mum and Dad went to the school to voice their displeasure to the principal about me being put into danger without anyone checking on my well-being. I didn't get an apology and neither did my parents. They just got told that there were an awful lot of children in the school, making it impossible to know where each child was at any particular moment. From what my parents told me, the school implied that I should have been able to keep up with my classmates.

We moved shortly after the incident and I eventually put the ordeal behind me. Unfortunately, it did make me more apprehensive around trails. To this day, I sometimes feel panicked when I walk along a trail even when I am with someone else.

I never got any sort of diagnosis as a child for my physical struggles, that would not come for many decades. I told myself that it was okay to be crap at sports because literally no one ever wanted me on their team anyway. Now the younger me couldn't possibly have any idea that the current me would end up seeing physical activity as my lifeline—my rescue from years of agony and anguish. The tables would turn.

Crash and Burn

I was in my teenage years, when I got into a bad car accident. I was driving home from seeing Kim, and didn't have a care in the world. It was late in the afternoon, but not quite rush hour. Driving along, my thoughts turned to almost being home. I had driven past this exact spot countless times before, as it was the same route I used getting back and forth to work.

There was a bend coming up, and the angle of my approach blocked the view of any traffic ahead. At that very moment, a car was waiting to make a left-hand turn onto a small side street. By the time I saw it, it was already too late to avoid a collision. I pumped my brakes as hard as I could trying to stop, but my actions couldn't avoid what was about to happen. I held the steering wheel tightly and prepared for impact. I was young and didn't realize that bracing likely contributed to the severity of my injuries.

I remained conscious, but knew instantly that I wasn't going to be able to get out of the car to exchange insurance details with the driver that I had hit. It was my first car accident and it was a doozy.

I didn't know exactly what injuries I had, but I could tell by the amount of pain that I was in, that I wasn't going to be going to work anytime soon. There were people coming up to the car asking if I was alright, they said that an ambulance was on the way. I was lucky that an ambulance had arrived quickly. This was before the days when everyone had a cell phone with them. Someone living on the side road must have heard the impact and called for help.

Upon arrival at the hospital, I was taken for X-rays, which confirmed the fact that I had fractured my right knee and my left wrist. I was too young to sign any surgical consent papers, so I had to wait for my Mum and Dad to come to the hospital. I was pretty groggy by the time they got there, but I put on my bravest face as they squeezed my hand and reassured me everything was going to be fine.

The next thing I remember was waking up in the hospital on the surgical recovery ward feeling very disoriented. I tried to get something from the nightstand beside me, but couldn't reach it because my leg was in a sling hooked up to a pulley system that was coming from a bar above me. My leg was laying there motionless, making it impossible for me to turn over.

It was extremely difficult to position myself in just the right spot to get any degree of comfort, and the comfort never lasted long. I lay with my leg suspended for a few days before any attempt was made to get me out of bed.

Kim always remembers his first visit with me after the crash, I went to give him a big hug and the cast on my wrist almost knocked him out cold. We had been together the day before without a care in the world. It is true what they say about life's ability to change at any moment. I was about to receive my first grown-up lesson regarding the power of the human spirit.

I can't remember the exact number of days I was in the hospital, but it was quite a while. I remember the bruises being really black and taking forever to change colour. I was a frightful sight for anyone walking into the room.

I would hold out for as long as I could before asking for pain medication, and was quite proud of my efforts. I routinely went past the time I needed to, before asking for more. As a teenager, I thought I knew everything, and was in grin-and-bear it mode. I didn't know that when you let medication deplete in your system before getting your next dose, your body has to work much harder to ease the pain level. Once the nurse told me that I was going too long and making it harder on myself, I had a rethink of my tactics. Lesson learned.

When the day came to learn how to use crutches, I really struggled. I had two physiotherapists trying to help, one on each side of me. I was a mess. I couldn't put any weight on my left side because of the broken wrist. The left side needed to be able to support me because the right side had the broken knee. I didn't think there was a workable solution. It was only at that moment that I realized how arduous my immediate future was going to be. There was going to be no quick fix.

The therapists were accustomed to finding ways around a situation so weren't thrown by my limitations. I ended up having two different crutches. A regular crutch on one side and one that was waist height that my arm slipped through for the side with the broken wrist. It looked really peculiar but I didn't have a choice if I wanted to get home. As I had always struggled with balance, relying on two sticks that I leaned on at different heights was next to impossible to get my head around.

After my accident, I had a long road of rehabilitation before me. Thinking of what lay ahead was going to get me nowhere. It would just get me frustrated and depressed. Instead, I tackled each day as a fresh start. It was my willpower alone that allowed me to take those first tentative moves that were more of a shuffle than a step. My body was reluctant to hold its own weight. It was a big deal to make it from my hospital bed to the chair just a few feet away. It was as though I had run a marathon, rather than stumble a few feet. I was completely exhausted after each effort.

Once I was able to make it out of my hospital room and down the corridor, my doctor was pleased enough with my progress to send me home, but only for a few weeks. The plan was that once my swelling had had a chance to go down and I was sufficiently recovered at home, I would be admitted to a rehabilitation hospital for intense in-patient physiotherapy.

It was boring not being able to do much, but healing at home was the easy part. Mum and Dad spoiled me. Dad would bring home bags of green grapes which were a personal favourite, and Mum made all of my favourite meals. Once I got to the rehab hospital the work really began. My pilot light was in for its biggest challenge to date.

I was in a room with three other people, Heather, Cindy, and Bernice. Heather was a young girl of about twelve. She was opposite me, in the bed closest to the window. She had been there for a long time before I arrived. Heather had severe rheumatoid arthritis and was confined to a wheelchair. Her bedsheets were silk because she couldn't stand the weight of regular hospital bedding. The silk also made it easier for her to get comfortable once she was in bed. Someone had crocheted her a really pretty lightweight bedspread making her corner of the room look cheery and less institutional. You could tell, just by looking at how she had her space decorated, that she wasn't going home anytime soon.

She was a pretty young thing with long light brown hair that her parents would brush as they would visit with her. Her smile was infectious. Over the coming days, just seeing how well she coped with everything that she was dealing with, put things clearly into perspective for me. My trials and tribulations felt insignificant in comparison.

Cindy was the lady directly opposite me, she was probably in her mid-thirties, and like me, she was recovering from surgery, what that surgery was I don't remember. What I do clearly remember, however, is that Cindy had only a partially formed ear on one side. If you just had a quick look at her, you may not notice right away, but once you knew it was there, it was the first thing that your eyes were drawn to. It was a birth defect; she had the top part of an ear and then it tapered off. The earlobe, such as it was, was ornamental. She was born without an ear canal and only had one functioning ear.

Being polite, for the first few days when I talked to her, I wouldn't allow myself to look in the direction of the partial ear, I focused just on the ear that she could hear out of. That soon subsided though and I started to talk to her just the way that I talked to anyone else.

This only left the lady directly beside me. Bernice was an elderly lady, but then as a teenager, everyone over 30 seemed old to me. She could have been anywhere from her sixties to her nineties it was impossible to tell. She had survived a house fire but sustained terrible burns everywhere that I could see. Her face, arms, and legs were nothing but burn scars. The nurses were needing to give her a great deal of attention. She wasn't going home anytime soon either. The curtains were almost always drawn around her hospital bed. Of the four of us, I was one of the lucky ones. It might take a long time, but I was going to get better.

The cause of Bernice's ordeal was falling asleep with a lit cigarette. I couldn't begin to imagine what she must have gone through, my heart went out to her.

We were in the late 1970s, and the hospital made allowances for patients who were smokers, if they couldn't get up, they could smoke in their beds. The only one of us who smoked was Bernice. Knowing the damage cigarettes had done to her, I simply assumed that she was no longer smoking, but I was wrong. One day we smelled smoke and realized that Bernice had a cigarette in her mouth and looked like she was about to pass out. All three of us pushed our call bells simultaneously. We needed help fast.

During the day whenever we were back in our rooms, we were always on alert in case it happened again. If I was in bed my only view of her was through the small slit in the curtains that separated us. If I wanted to check if things were okay for myself, I had to grab the bed rails and twist my bad leg in her direction, this hurt a lot so I only did it when the suspense had gotten too much to bear. All three of us were scared to go to sleep, or even close our eyes. We were sitting ducks if a fire broke out. At night my thoughts would flit between what I had to do to physically get better, and what if I fell asleep and was burned to death.

Every attempt to calm myself down was futile. I hadn't thought of death before and certainly would have no reason to think of my own mortality were it not for the fact I was lying beside my potential killer. Kim's Mum would constantly tell me that everything is meant, but I questioned her logic when it came to my current situation.

Until this point in time, I had always relied on logic to maintain my positive outlook. I thought my way through a situation. Having been brought up in a religious household, I had my beliefs, but thought what was the point of praying? Prayers were for things like world peace, no amount of "Please God," was going to stop Bernice from smoking.

The nurses always put my bed rails up whenever I was in bed, it made it easier to reposition myself. In an emergency though, what chance did I have to get out of bed, get my mismatched crutches and get out of there? I could barely walk unassisted and running was impossible. I had nightmares of being trapped in a fire and ending up like Bernice or dead.

Heather couldn't get out of bed without help. In a fire, she had no hope of getting into a wheelchair and wheeling herself to safety in time. We were in the danger zone. In all, Bernice almost fell asleep three times while smoking, with me trapped in the bed just a few feet away. This was a ridiculous situation to be in. Someone had to stop Bernice from getting anywhere near a cigarette.

After the third incident, the hospital staff finally came to their senses and moved the three of us elsewhere in the hospital. They also confiscated Bernice's lighter and cigarettes.

My days were very structured at the hospital. Monday to Friday, I would have physiotherapy throughout the day, with short breaks for rest and lunch. The only easy sessions were the ones for my wrist. I would put my hand in a warm vat of liquid wax and let the heat penetrate my wrist. It felt surprisingly good, and I didn't actually have to do anything. This was in sharp contrast to what I had to do to get my leg mobile again.

Clearly, walking was my biggest hurdle. I got the same physiotherapist each day. She was lovely: she was part doctor, part taskmaster and part cheerleader all rolled into one. Progress was painfully slow. Each degree I gained in my range of motion was a monumental feat.

I couldn't stay in the hospital forever and didn't want to. On the weekends, there was no physiotherapy, nothing happened. I called them the wasted days. The only highlight was the visiting hours from 3 to 8. Kim visited as often as he could, but he was working as a bellman at the time, which meant that he worked quite a few night shifts. I didn't get to see him then, so I worked as hard as I could while he was gone, so that I could show him how far I had progressed whenever he came to see me.

After the accident, my singular focus was to get my life back on track, nothing else mattered. I spend hours working on each boring detail, running through my exercises, rest and repeat. I was relentless.

I know a lot of people, when injured, automatically go to physiotherapy as part of their recovery. They don't do the work that they are supposed to do between visits and then complain that they didn't fully regain the movement that they had lost. If that person was honest with themselves, they know full well that it's not the therapist's fault at all. The fault is theirs.

I have spent many hours in rehab facilities over the years trying to recover from various fractures. It hurts and it's hard, pure and simple. There isn't really any way to make it fun —at least none that I have found. Horrible or not, I always have done the work. If you think that the therapists can't tell that you decided to skip the recommended exercise to do something you enjoy instead, you are just fooling yourself.

The way that I see it, people like physiotherapists and other health-care specialists show you what to do to get better and how to do it properly. At the end of their work day, they go home to their families and private lives. If I don't want to do the work, it isn't really going to change their lives any. But if I listen and do the work the way they have shown me to,

I could be changing my life. So why then would I not put in the work?

It took about three months to recover before I felt I had gotten things working as well as I could expect. I never managed to get my knee to work the way it had but there came a point when no amount of rehab would give me more mobility, and I knew I would just have to accept that this was as good as it was going to get for now.

Stairs remained difficult, you use different muscles depending on whether you are going up or down. Neither direction is particularly easy. I need something to hold onto. There are certain pitches of stairs that work better than others, but for the most part, as long as there is a handrail I can manage, even if it means going one step at a time.

I now have about a six-inch scar that goes horizontally across my knee. The scar, over time, has faded, back then it was red and ugly. Wearing a dress only drew attention to it. I liked wearing dresses though so just kept doing it. Periodically I still get strangers feeling compelled to pass judgment on my scar, I look upon my scars as battle wounds—they are unintended souvenirs of battles well-fought. It no longer matters to me what people think. They can provide comments or stay silent. I am a combination of my life experiences, and nothing is going to hold me back unless I let it.

About seven years after the original surgery, when my knee began to feel that it was going to give out. I discovered that I had not had my knee cap completely removed as I had always believed. I still had half a knee cap which now wasn't staying in place.

I was sent to an orthopedic surgeon who assured me that he could perform a routine surgery that would rectify that situation. I agreed to the surgery which ended up being among the biggest regrets off my life.

Instead of removing what was left of my knee cap, he rearranged all of my muscles to hold my partial kneecap in the wrong place. I was never the same again physically after that surgery. Top it off, he didn't make my incision neat and tidy. I was horrified when I discovered I now had an even longer scar going down my leg in addition to the one going across it. Like a permanent bull's eye, I now had a giant plus sign on my right leg. That's why I refer to my right now as my positive side.

I was back seeing a physiotherapist several times a week. Going through the familiar exercise routine to get my knee working. Unlike before, I wasn't making headway and was facing months of rehabilitation.

Sometimes, knowing what to expect is not a positive thing. I couldn't trick myself into believing this was going to be easy. I knew better than that, I'd been down this road before, but that didn't help matters. I was seven years older than last time, and trying to get already damaged body parts to recover was a momentous challenge.

Although I gave it my best efforts and positive spin, I was losing ground. I knew things weren't right, but getting someone to listen took a few years. Periodically I broached the subject with whomever my family doctor was at the time but kept getting brushed off. I never managed to get past his office.

One day at work, one of my colleagues was talking to me and said: "You can't go on like this, you need to do something about it." With that, she gave me the name of an orthopedic surgeon. He was a sports injury specialist. I didn't get injured playing sports, but this fellow was the team doctor for the provincial professional hockey team, he had to be top-notch if they were using him, Canadians take hockey very seriously. If he was good enough for professional hockey he was good enough for me.

One of the first things he said to me when we met was that he knew exactly what my problem was. He could see the issue clearly from the X-rays I had brought with me. My muscles weren't where they were meant to be, and they were holding my knee cap in the wrong place.

That explained things but now what? He said he couldn't get things as good as new, but he could make things significantly better than they were. It wasn't a quick fix. Surgery was scheduled a few short weeks after the appointment to remove my patella fragment.

The surgery went extremely well. I was becoming a professional when it came to knowing what to do post-surgery, so there were no surprises. The thing with chronic injuries is that it takes a toll on you mentally. It is a lot easier to have positivity for a defined length of time than it is to remain positive year in and year out, without any end date.

It was a case of deja-vu whenever the issue of my knee demanded attention. I had been down that road too many times before. I knew better than to simply do nothing, physically I knew the drill. It has been the mental component that unfortunately doesn't have an automatic reset button.

The human body is a miraculous work of art but if anything is out of whack then nothing seems to go right. Mentally and physically, I have to be in sync before I can feel healthy. My pilot light is a critical component of achieving my successes so I nurture the flame every chance I get.

The Pilot Light Effect

A Change of Direction

My work life had always felt solid. After nearly 30 years it was entrenched in who I was. I felt valued and respected and thoroughly enjoyed what I did for a living. My work involved contact with many people from all walks of life and I thrived. I was happy to go to work each day. I took my work seriously.

The company I worked for had an annual award of excellence that had begun about five years before I was a recipient. I was honoured, as there were not many awards given. I had gotten my health back, work was going well, and life felt storybook perfect. Little did I know that night at the awards gala that within three months I would be fighting for my job along with hundreds of people, many of whom I had worked alongside for decades. What happened in those few months made the excellence award meaningless to me. I had gotten a lovely bracelet that matches the ring I got for my twenty-five years of service with the award money I received. Both of them now sit in my jewelry box, where they have been ever since I left the company.

It was a pivotal moment that I hadn't prepared for. First, there was the shock element. Our office was all sent into a meeting, late on a Friday afternoon, with big-wigs from head office who had flown in for the occasion. We listened quietly as they began detailing the sharp change of direction that the company was taking. We were praised for our years of service. It soon became apparent, however, that we were not going to be the face of the company going forward.

I started working for them three weeks after my high school graduation. I didn't know anything else. I reassured myself that a lot of skills were transferable and continually gave myself pep talks when I thought I needed one. My biggest concern was that there were going to be hundreds of people all with the same skill sets applying for work elsewhere. There was nothing that I could do about that fact. I needed to stand out, but how?

We were given some heavy-duty sales quotas to meet and our managers began booking times to sit with each of us to listen to our phone calls in the name of "education," their job was to improve customer service by teaching us to up-sell products and features more effectively. I wasn't about to give people something that they didn't want, I wasn't hired for that. I know things change, but feeling as though you have to hard-sell everyone all of the time wasn't sitting well with me.

What started to happen once the quota requirement took full effect was, as soon as some people realized they could not get a sale out of the call, mysteriously the call would somehow be disconnected. The customer would phone back hopping mad, and who could blame them. Now you had the quotas and time restrictions to contend with as well as an angry customer that wanted to be able to vent. It wasn't everyone that was dropping calls, but these were desperate times and desperate measures. Our livelihoods were on the line.

In my department, we were given almost impossible targets to meet and these targets would change part way through the month. This ensured that a certain percentage of people failed. If you did not meet the monthly target, you got a letter stating that you were unsatisfactory. If you received three of these notices, we were told that the company would have grounds to fire you based on your performance. The stress was through the roof. I don't know if they could actually do that but I, like everyone else, didn't want to find out.

Our jobs were being primarily outsourced to the Philippines and India. The positions available in Canada would be limited. I could accept a job in another province but there would still be quotas. I could move there and still end up losing my job. I was hanging on by a thread by this point. I don't know one person that wasn't on the edge of tears at some point while all this nonsense was going on.

My mind went to dark places that I never thought my mind was capable of. I didn't tell a living soul but I would lay awake worrying about going to work. Not just the pressure of targets and dealing with difficult people, but would I make it through the day? Surely this can't continue, I had two choices, stay or go. I had a talk with Kim, fighting back the tears, I said that I had given it my best shot, but I couldn't go on with the way things were at work. It just wasn't healthy. He agreed and assured me that he was right behind me if I wanted to leave, all I had to do was accept the package offered and walk away.

I went into the office the next day and sent my boss an e-mail saying that I would accept the package. The decision had been a hard one but I would be accepting the severance package. A wonderful 27-year career had come down to this moment. It wasn't the way I had imagined leaving a job that I previously loved.

I couldn't believe it when I discovered that saying you wanted the package wasn't a guarantee that you would get it. The company would then advise you if you got the package and when you could leave. First, they made it horrible to stay, now they were making it hard to go.

I got my first unsatisfactory performance letter three days before I was due to leave in the middle of August. When I saw what my manager was handing me, I lost my cool and vented my displeasure. I didn't yell but I certainly was acting out of character. The happy-go-lucky me was nowhere in sight. It had felt like a character assassination. I took it personally and was on the warpath. The only reason I had not made their foolish quota was that I had been pulled off of my regular assignment to help elsewhere. They didn't take that into consideration.

I told my boss how wrong she was to have given me the letter. She tried to make me feel better by assuring me that everyone knew what a good employee I was. Yes, I agreed, but now I have it in writing that I am unsatisfactory. In my over twenty-seven-year career, I had never gotten a poor performance review. Now my parting gift was this stinking letter stating that I was unsatisfactory. It made me feel worthless.

A person could be excused for thinking we were all in the

same boat, when in actual fact we were all in the same storm, however, we were each navigating our own boats and making choices based on how the impact of the restructuring effected us personally. Someone in a different office committed suicide, and I know other people had tried. Is any job worth your life? All this in the name of corporate advancement. One life gone is one life too many.

Fortunately looking back now years later, I don't dwell on that time. People move on and heal. The company had been good to me for decades. It was just that last few months that were hell. They are still in business, bigger than ever. It is now just a part of their corporate history. Nothing more than a moment in time. That moment in time changed how I look at things. It took away some of the innocence that I had about people, about the world being fair, and that the good guys always win. They don't always win, they become survivalists.

My pilot light had taken a beating. It felt as though I had just been in a boxing ring and lost the fight. By the time I left, I felt disoriented and that I didn't belong anywhere. I was out of the situation now, but my body hadn't learned how to let go of being in a constant fight or flight scenario yet.

I went into hibernation for the first couple of months. It was unsettling to be out of the habit of simply getting up and going to work each day. I missed the people. I missed being good at what I did. Above all, I hated not contributing to the household finances. There is only so much personal house cleaning any human can do.

Kim never pressured me to find work, he was great. He didn't want to move to a different province either. He reassured me that we would be just fine, and I knew that he was right. He was confident that I would find work once I felt more settled.

I am not good at the whole poor me thing. I needed to allow myself to put the whole thing behind me, and embrace this new chapter that I had been thrust into. I had done some self-care in the early days. I visited family and got more in tune with things that mattered. I embraced my hobbies and met friends for lunch. Nothing startling, but I could feel the real me starting to show herself again, and it felt good. My pilot light started to regain its glow. instead of waiting to see what happened next and reacting to it. I took control. My pilot light shines its brightest when I take control.

I decided that for the time being, I just wanted a job rather than a career. It would put me back into the job market, have me contributing to the household finances, along with seeing people and feeling more productive. For now, a simple job would tick all of the boxes. My plan was to look at career paths in the coming months and go from there. I found a part-time job just a couple of miles from home. It wasn't going to be a forever thing. For now, though it was perfect.

Gone was my dental and medical plan. We still had a bit of coverage from Kim's work but it wasn't at the level that I had been accustomed to. I figured we were both young enough that nothing bad should happen. A crystal ball would have been good, but none of us know what lays ahead.

Things went on as life always does. Before long, my

temporary job was more long-term than I had anticipated. Work liked me as an employee, I was happy enough, getting raises regularly, and working as many hours as I wanted to. Despite my best efforts I never managed to get a full-time position with the company. That irked me, but not enough to do anything about it.

I had started to think that this was the time to either secure full-time employment where I was, or start looking elsewhere for something more fulfilling. My life decisions are never spontaneous. I am a cautious soul at the best of times. I tend to think things through thoroughly before I take action. I was at one of those points in my life when I was blissfully unaware of a plot twist ahead.

A Downward Spiral

It all began on what seemed to be an ordinary workday. I had just finished a lovely vacation with family who was visiting us from England. I was ready to get back into my routine. My job involved me standing all day, and the anti-fatigue mats provided had always done the trick up until now. Suddenly out of the blue I got a swift stabbing pain in my left leg, I just thought that my body was protesting about being back at work after having a month off. I didn't even give as much as a second thought to what I would later discover was a colossal warning of impending doom.

The pain subsided as quickly as it came. It was a jarring pain, deep within my thigh that traveled down my leg, and it happened a few more times throughout my shift that day. It was sharp enough that I wanted to cry but swift enough that tears never had a chance to form. I didn't even tell Kim about it when I got home. I figured it was an isolated incident.

Over the next week or so, there were a few more pain zaps, swift but mighty. I only seemed to get the pain while I was at work, so I thought about what the trigger could be. Was I standing poorly? Do I need to look at working shorter shifts, or perhaps space out my days off? Once the pain didn't go away on its own, I knew that I needed to do something about it. I told Kim and then made an appointment to see my doctor.

I had had the same doctor for several years. He was well aware that I only went to see him when I had a genuine medical concern. He listened quietly and took it all in. He examined my feet and legs, then confidently stated that orthotics should do the trick. He referred me to a movement rehabilitation facility and I waited patiently for the appointment date to arrive. The wait ended up being several weeks, and my situation worsened. Those shooting pains were now up both of my legs and into my feet —and far more frequent.

By the time I got into the orthotics appointment, the person taking an imprint of my feet had a hell of a time touching them. My feet have always been extremely sensitive to touch. I instantly pull away, because my feet clench so tight, it is a miracle that any blood flows to them at all. Honestly, it is a knee-jerk reaction that I am unable to control. I don't even like touching my own feet, never mind letting anyone else do it. That day I had no choice, though, my pain levels were through the roof. It took everything in me to let him hold my feet. He ended up getting an additional colleague to help, and two people at once was torture. I tried to co-operate as best that I could. My mind was willing, but my body certainly wasn't. I couldn't wait to get out of there.

I thought that everyone's feet clenched to the touch and that the toes were meant to curl. I never had any reason to study other people's feet. I didn't see what is now blatantly obvious, that people's feet are generally flat and toes are straight. I have a high arch and my feet feel as though they are being pulled inward. It's no wonder my feet hurt. I used to get terrible cramps in my legs growing up. They were put down as growing pains at the time and nothing more was done. A childhood doctor had recommended I strengthen my foot muscles by trying to pick up a pencil with my toes. I couldn't get the toes to unclench long enough to wrap around a pencil, never mind pick it up.

The orthotics arrived: they were black, square, and boxy with thick velcro straps. I aged myself by 30 years each time I put them on. They were without question the ugliest footwear known to man. All I needed was some white hair and glasses and I could have easily become my own grandmother. Isn't it bad enough to need orthotics, without them stripping away any hope of appearing attractive? Where is the dignity? I had never spent so much on a pair of shoes before in my entire life and it took everything I had not to immediately toss the horrible things in the bin. I know high heels were out of the question, but surely to God, there had to be something between high heels and these hideous foot anchors.

Despite the fact that I loathed the shoes, I wore them religiously. But there was no improvement whatsoever; in fact, things were getting worse. The stabbing pains in the legs continued, close to constant at this point and increasing with intensity. How, where, and when the pains would happen remained a mystery. I knew that I would get intense pain somewhere but that was all I knew for sure.

The pain would be under my toes as though someone was sticking a sharp poker under my toenails at one moment, or using an electric drill to penetrate my ankle bone without anesthetic the next. It didn't matter if I was just taking it easy, doing something fun with my friends, keeping myself busy at work or at home watching TV. Whatever I was doing physically didn't have any impact on the situation.

When I broke my knee, the physiotherapist had given me a set of exercises that I did faithfully. I took the medication as directed, would ice my knee if it began to swell, and rested as needed. The list of do's and don'ts was straightforward. I had a clear road map to recovery. For this though, I had nothing.

Up to this point, the pain had only affected my legs. I had no reason to believe that the pain would spread elsewhere, but it did. I remember the day when I began having difficulty with my hands. Kim and I were out one morning and he was holding my hand as we walked. I could feel my hand ache, as though he was holding too tightly. It was a knee-jerk reaction to pull away.

"What's the matter?" he asked.

"You are hurting me," I replied.

I figured I could simply change hands and carry on. The other side was better, but I just kept asking him to hold on lighter and lighter. At some point we thought, what's the point? My hand was just sort of laying on top of his.

That probably doesn't seem like a big deal to most people, but we both knew that I needed to hold hands for stability. I did let go for a few minutes, but I couldn't tell you who was more nervous about the whole thing. Kim kept looking expecting me to fall and trying to be ready. It was all a bit too much. I took his hand as lightly as I could and didn't say another word.

Kim has always looked out for me. He changed things as needed as my downward spiral continued. If we were going downstairs and there were no handrails, he would be right beside me. Depending on the pitch, he would go before me, standing on each step as I would hold onto his shoulders and ease my way down each step. His body being ahead of me would stop me from falling should I start to wobble forward. If I was going up the stairs, he would be behind me just in case I tipped backward unexpectedly.

With that kind of help required, you can understand how I could stress over being on my own. Being out alone is something that fit people take for granted. It wasn't that Kim was enabling me to stay unfit, he was lovingly trying to keep me safe.

It wasn't constant pain with the hands at first, but then that was exactly how the pain had started in my leg. I started to wonder where it was going to show up next. It was taking over my body as well as my thoughts. Each jolt of pain felt as though I was being probed with an electrode. They were multiple simultaneous electric shocks. The pain was horrendous.

The orthotics were definitely doing nothing for me. When the time came I was thrilled to be rid of them. I wouldn't have been so quick to be filled with glee had I known what was just around the corner.

Medical Misery

Because there had been such difficulty getting the imprint for my orthotics I had asked at the clinic when I was there, what my next step would be should the orthotics fail to provide relief. I wasn't wishing for failure, it simply seemed a little too easy a fix for something that I thought was developing into a serious situation. They had recommended that I be referred to a physiatrist. I had never heard of such a specialist. I later discovered that their area of expertise is referred to as physical medicine specializing in movement, the explanation of what a physiatrist does make some limited sense to me. Perhaps this will be the person that makes all my physical problems disappear. I certainly hoped so.

I never seem to get the easy fixes. I had given the orthotics a good try, but it was obvious to me that we needed to do something else. This didn't surprise me, as I had never put much faith into orthotics being the fix. I was just going along with anything the doctors suggested. I had no idea what direction I needed to go, but I had to try something different than what I was doing. Time was marching on. My pain continued to worsen, and I had to take action. I went back to the doctor, updated him on what had transpired, and asked to be referred to a physiatrist.

I usually went to my appointments by myself. I couldn't expect Kim to take time off from work to come with me whenever I needed to see a specialist. For the physiatrist appointment, my friend Sue offered to come with me. More often than not I would find myself waiting at least an hour or more in the waiting room to see any doctor, so I thought it would be nice to pass the time with a friend there for a change. Sue and I had been the closest of friends for over 20 years at this point in time. She was eager to find out what was wrong with me, as well.

The physiatrist was connected to the same rehabilitation facility I had gone to for the orthotics. This turned out to be beneficial as he had access to the records of my appointment and knew the difficulty the two technicians had had casting for my footwear, without me needing to explain the whole ordeal to him.

I waited months for my appointment. I was intrigued about what a physiatrist would do. As his expertise was movement, I thought he could point out what was causing the pain and correct it quickly. I was confident that all it was going to take was for me to explain my symptoms, he would have the answer, suggest a few things, put my mind at rest and send me on my merry way.

The doctor was nice, quite young, but old enough to have experience behind him. He was a man of few words. It was more of a question period. I found it hard to explain in detail what was going on with me physically, as I didn't understand it myself. I didn't have just one spot that was hurting. I felt a little foolish saying sometimes it hurts here, but other times it hurts there. How could the pain in my hands be related to the fact that my leg hurt. I could see the leg and feet might be related but certainly not all 3 it didn't make sense to me, but I hoped that it would make sense to him.

We chatted briefly, and then he said that he needed to do a nerve conduction test. I didn't know what a nerve conduction test was, but if it meant finding answers, I was completely on board with having the procedure. By the way that he was talking, it sounded like it was no big deal—not legalized torture.

He never fully explained to my satisfaction what was about to happen. He simply asked me to lay on the examination table where I was connected to a machine that had electrodes. These electrodes were placed at strategic points along my arms and legs. It was at this point that he advised that he would send an electrical current through the electrodes and measure the nerves' reaction to the current. He didn't even think to warn me that this test was excruciatingly painful. It certainly would have helped prepare me a little.

Oh my GOD!!! The places in my body where I would normally get my neurological zaps became hyper-attentive the very second that the testing began. Each time the pulse happened, my nerves convulsed. The impulses surged through my body every 10-15 seconds or so. No sooner would I survive a blast then the next one would come. It was like being caught out in an electrical storm in the middle of a field holding nothing but a metal sign saying "here I am." It hurt like hell.

As if that wasn't bad enough, he kept increasing the intensity as we went along. I was crawling on the ceiling by the time the test was concluded. It felt like it lasted for hours when in reality it was maybe 30 minutes. As far as I was concerned that was 30 minutes too long.

The entire time I was shrieking on the inside, "Make it stop, make it stop." I would have been more outwardly vocal, but the last thing I wanted to do was risk giving him any possible reason to start the test over again from the beginning. I knew I wouldn't be able to survive it a second time. I had barely survived the first one.

Once the test was over, I was left alone to recover for a few minutes while he went to analyze my results. I couldn't move. I was in pain that up to that point I had never experienced before in my entire life, not even when I had broken my knee cap. The nerves were pulsating angrily, waging war on me. The neurological jabs were relentless. The machine might be disconnected now, but no one had told my body to stop reacting—it had a mind of its own.

When he returned, in his best clinical voice, he told me that I should not let anyone talk me into orthotics.

"It's too late for that sage bit of advice," I thought.

He said that the problem had nothing to do with my feet, but the problem was either in my spine or in my brain. Whoa, where is the audiologist? I couldn't possibly have been hearing him correctly.

The shock of his words and immense pain from the testing made the rest of what he had to say just too much to take in. He said he would send a letter with his recommendations to my family doctor, who would take it from there.

When we were done, I can remember thanking him on my way back out to his reception area. Imagine that! Thanking someone for doing something horrendous to you. I had lost my mind. The procedure had me more unbalanced than usual. I had difficulty walking straight, feeling quite disoriented. I think that I can now understand why a prizefighter seems like they are all over the place after a match. My body had gone into the ring and was now paying the price.

Sue said I was as white as a ghost when she saw me come through the door. I told her what had happened and where he thought my problem was, but after that, I just couldn't find the words to talk. Sue was so alarmed by my condition that she didn't know what to do. Should she take me to the emergency department or take me home? I had had enough of doctors for one day, so I really wanted to go home. She was reluctant, but Sue did eventually agree to take me home as I requested. The ride was the quietest one that we had ever shared together.

She walked me to my front door and normally would have come on in. Whenever things are bad for either of us, we just make ourselves a cup of tea, have a good chat, and then formulate a plan. If we can't get a plan to come together, we just listen to one another. Ours is a simple, perfect friendship. This time I didn't even want tea, that never happens. That's a bright red flag for anyone who knows me. Although Sue didn't want to leave me alone, I didn't give her a choice, I told her to go. All I wanted to do was to crawl into bed. At that point, I wouldn't have even cared if I had died during the night. I was so worn out. I was on information overload and it was all I could do just to breathe.

It took months for the nerves to stop twitching and revert back to the pain levels I had been experiencing before the test. It felt like a massive step backward. I had been suffering for so long, I couldn't work much and everyday living was a chore. I endured the nerve conduction test to get some answers. But I only had more questions.

The fact that something could be wrong with my spine or brain kept me awake at night. My thoughts went to darker places. What if I don't get to live to old age? If anyone suggests surgery, should I contemplate it or flat out refuse? What if I said yes and something went wrong? I would be screwing up my entire life and Kim's as well. I would only have myself to blame. I don't think that I could live with that. I was thankful for the escape from my thoughts once my medications took effect. The medication always made me sleepy. That sleep was the only escape from the thoughts that were consuming me.

I was digging a bigger and bigger hole for myself, one that I couldn't see getting myself out of, even with Kim's help. I wasn't used to not being in control. No amount of wishful thinking would help. I would need some educated allies.

As my health declined, I needed more and more medical devices. I had so many mobility aids that I swear that I could have started my own rental shop, except for the sad fact that I needed all the gadgets myself. At one time or another, there have been grab bars strategically placed throughout the house, in addition to walkers, crutches, wheelchairs, and even commodes. Knee braces, the aforementioned orthotics, compression socks. Let's not forget the bed rail so that I could pull myself out of bed, or the long step I had beside the bed because I didn't have the range of motion to get myself onto the bed without it.

If someone was clearing out my house and didn't know me, they would probably believe they were in the home of an 80- or 90-year-old. I would have been in my late forties or early fifties at the time, and aging rapidly.

On occasion I would find myself thinking about Bernice, wondering if I could safely get out of the house quickly if there was a fire or another emergency. Was I any safer now than I was when I was in the hospital bed beside her all those years ago? If I was being honest, I don't think so.

Stump the Specialists

I had to switch family physicians after my original family doctor retired. Fortunately, he had sold his practice rather than just closing it. Thank heavens I did not fall through the cracks, with only a local walk-in clinic left to go to for help. My medical needs had become far too complex to rely on a 10-minute appointment with a stranger. How could I condense my story down to 10 minutes? It couldn't be done.

It takes a while to get comfortable with a new doctor. I was impressed with him, though, right from my first appointment. Dr. Welsh* is a tall, slender man, with a very professional manner. My first impression was that he was a perfect blend of quiet, reserved, methodical and caring, without getting too emotionally involved.

My medical file is on the large side. I was a couple of years into my saga by the point I met Dr. Welsh. The thought of starting over with someone else was daunting. I found that just talking about my health was emotionally and physically exhausting. I had to put all that aside. It was critical that I build a rapport with him because I needed him.

When we met for the first time, I liked the fact that I hadn't been put into an examination room to wait for him. When it came to my time to see him, he came out to the waiting area and called out my name. He then greeted me warmly and led me into his office. I thought that the receptionist had just been busy to do that for him, but I was wrong, he did that on every visit. He says it gives him great insight into how people are feeling by simply watching how they get up and come towards him. That one gesture stood out to me. I had been seeing a lot of doctors, all of whom had their own approach. He was the only one to come out of his office and welcome me. He was standing out already.

He quickly looked through the paperwork he had in the file. What he read was just the most current information about me. I learned later that I had more than just one file. He then asked if I didn't mind, would I come back in a week's time. He wanted to take my files home to read, away from any work distractions. There was a lot of information to go through and he really needed to understand what was going on. When I came back, we would go through everything together, he would do a full check-up and we would go from there.

He assured me that at any time, if I needed to speak to him, I could call and leave word with his receptionist and he would call me back at the end of the day. If I needed to see him, he would make time for me. What more could I have asked for?

The appointment went much better than I had anticipated. He came across as human, and someone that I could talk to. Those are perfect characteristics for a doctor. We were going to get along just fine, I could tell. Already he had me feeling at ease just in those first few minutes. When you see a doctor as often as I was, being at ease was essential.

Once Dr. Welsh was in charge, medical appointments with specialists became a bit of a blur. He had breathed new life into finding a solution for me. It had given me renewed hope. After the physiatrist, I met with a rheumatologist, acupuncturist, and three neurologists. One was an ordinary neurologist, one was a neurosurgeon, and the third was a neurological professor. Pretty much if a doctor had an "ist" at the end of their title and their specialty even remotely pertained to my situation, I saw them.

With each appointment, I would go over the details of my current situation. Conditions changed over time, so although the basics remained the same, each doctor got a slightly different version of what I was experiencing because no two days were alike or even two hours. Without spending days going over the history of my deterioration, it was next to impossible for any doctor to jump in and have a clear understanding of what was going on. There wasn't a defined path to follow.

If you have a confirmed medical diagnosis, then you are referred to one specialist. That specialist knows what to do to treat you. There is a sense of structure. When you are still searching for a diagnosis and cure, you see so many people. Emotionally it is a peculiar sensation, swinging between hope and despair. You worry about what type of specialist you are due to see, not only worrying that you might have something sinister, but also what the treatment might look like to cure you.

Other times you hope that the next specialist will walk into the examination room surrounded by a halo of light because he/she was the one with the answer. Someone had to know something. Surely one human being can't possibly stump all of the specialists. I now related to the term "searching for a needle in a haystack" on a much more personal level.

At one point, I had myself convinced that I didn't care what it was that I ended up having, I just wanted someone to tell me what the problem was. Somehow my mindset had changed to the point that even a bad diagnosis was better than no diagnosis at all.

This state of limbo went on forever, so it was only natural that my pilot light was taking a beating. I waited months to see each specialist. If they had suggested trying something, it would involve a trial of a few months. I would embrace what they suggested, follow their recommendations to the letter. I contributed everything I could to ensure success. On those occasions that I had been offered a follow-up appointment, it was common for those to be booked six months away or even longer.

I was now years into this existence of endless pain and medical appointments. It didn't feel like I was any further ahead. The pain was causing me to do less and less, and I was on a downward trajectory. The less I did, the less that I was able to do. I had given up working and was now rarely leaving the house. Kim worked long hours, so I spent a great deal of time on my own with my thoughts and pain for company. I didn't have the energy to cry.

I had to make a conscious effort to have a good day. That at least managed to keep my pilot light lit, but it certainly took work just to keep that little spark from going out completely. If I didn't concentrate on at least trying to find happiness, it would be far too easy to wallow in my situation.

My best attempts to make each day a good one had some epic fails. That is inevitable, so whenever that happened, I gave myself a pretty good pep talk. Not everything in a bad day had to be bad. I looked for anything that was positive, and then went from there. My solution to keep my spark glowing was to feed it. To give it whatever joy and positivity I could find.

One guaranteed way for me to find joy was spending time embroidering. It not only brought me joy, but I could also see something beautiful being created. Each picture, depending on the complexity of the pattern, could easily take three or four hundred hours, or more to complete. I think all of my family have at least something that I have made for them. While I was stitching away it not only passed the time, I would think about the person that I was making it for, and what that person means to me. I found that by thinking of them as I went along, I was reminded that they were each invested in my recovery. They love me and wanted to see my sassy, fun-loving side return. Each embroidered piece is a labour of love.

I am glad that I made the most of the time I did spend embroidering because stitching became a victim of my deteriorating hands. It was something else that I added to the list of things that I could no longer do. It saddened me to see my treasure trove of embroidery supplies collecting dust. I couldn't bring myself to sell what I had though, I just had to hope that one day I could start it up again.

Kim and I made a choice not to talk about my medical condition often. We felt that neither of us could do anything about it, and we were just giving permission for the situation to take over our lives if we kept going on about it. It wasn't a case of sticking our heads in the sand. We knew that we needed to play the long game. Keep hope alive by all means, but we had to be realistic, this was potentially something that was always going to be with us. If that ended up being what happens we had to take decisive action not to let it rule our lives. Kim knew without asking how much pain I was in. He need only listen to my spontaneous outbursts when the neurological zaps had reached a point that I could no longer contain the scream for confirmation. We took each day as it came while we waited for a resolution.

My only consistent link to the medical field was Dr. Welsh. I could tell that he felt empathy for my situation. He was true to his word that he would leave no stone unturned. I felt, based on what the physiatrist said, that my greatest hope for an answer remained with the neurologists. I think that Dr. Welsh was on the same page. He would always wait for the assessments to come in, and then he would chart the course forward.

I thought it was a stroke of genius on his part when he arranged for me to be seen at a rapid assessment clinic at the hospital. It was a multi-hour appointment where I was subjected to a barrage of tests. It felt like they were looking at every possibility with fresh eyes. Not quite starting from scratch, but it was as though the cavalry had been called in.

It was at that clinic that I met a visiting associate neurological professor from a prominent university a few thousand miles away. He was on a one-year exchange program. I figured that luck was obviously changing in my favour. I would never normally have access to a neurological professor. I felt quite privileged to be given the opportunity to meet with him. I started to believe that if anyone would have an answer it would have to be him.

On the day of the assessment at the hospital, sixteen vials of blood were taken from me. The lab was being given lots to do and the various doctors that I was due to see had the results before my appointment time with them was done. They had a great system going. This was how I imagined speed-dating, except it wasn't potential dates it was doctors.

Two nights prior to seeing the professor, there had been a news program on the television talking about testing that had been developed in Europe. It had discovered a link between narrowing of the carotid artery in people with MS and other neurological issues. Kim and I had watched it because, if I found any program in the television guide that had anything to do with neurological conditions or improving health in general, it would become must-see TV for us.

Because this doctor was an associate professor of neurology, he was being inundated with calls from across the country. They were people from all walks of life asking to be tested. As luck would have it, he approached me while the technician was completing one of my other tests. He asked her if she knew what to look for when testing someone's carotid artery.

Because I was right there with the two of them, he used me (or more specifically my carotid artery) to demonstrate what she needed to do. I would have asked him about the program that I had seen, but as it turned out I didn't need to, he was already checking me for the condition that the program had been talking about. My carotid artery was fine. I was tested for something else obscure and passed and had a properly functioning carotid artery to prove it. That was a definite bonus. I was getting lots of peculiar tests done on me for some pretty out-there, medical conditions. One by one, culprits were very slowly being struck from the list of possible causes of my medical woes.

After the carotid artery excitement had finished, I explained to the doctor what was going on with me, he listened attentively and then left to analyze some results.

When he reappeared, he said that my MRI showed that there was something not quite right going on with my brain. Exactly what that was, he didn't elaborate. It had likely been from birth, a form of cerebral palsy, he said. Something he called Little's disease.

I had never heard of anything called Little's disease; I had heard the term cerebral palsy though but didn't know much about it. I was confused because my limited exposure to someone with cerebral palsy involved someone in a wheelchair who couldn't communicate. That wasn't me.

So what happens next? Now that I had a name, what do we need to do to fix this? The professor said I seemed like a very nice lady, but there really wasn't anything that could be done to alter my current situation. Although he never verbalized it, as far as I was concerned, he was telling me that I was going to be in pain until I died that was all there was to it.

This was not what I had been waiting years to hear. I had finally met the specialist that I didn't stump, only to hate what he had to say and the fact he could not provide a cure.

Not wanting to write me off entirely, he did arrange for me to have another MRI in three months' time in order to compare the results. He would be leaving within a few weeks of the second MRI, but I managed to squeeze in a final appointment with him back in his office just prior to his one-year term being finished when he would be gone for good.

On further investigation, after I had left the clinic, I discovered that cerebral palsy is a group of permanent movement disorders that appear in early childhood. It was then that the light went on. Symptoms often include poor coordination, yes, that is definitely me. Stiff weak muscles, yes, that's me too. As I went through the list, I had several of the symptoms listed to some varying degree. Oh my God, that explains so much. All those failed attempts to be good at sports. The cramping in my feet. Everything could fit into that diagnosis.

When a professor gives you the diagnosis you have been looking for, once you have it, you stop looking for other possibilities. When nothing can be done, you believe them.

I had one more shot with the professor before he was due to leave, and my appointment date was coming up soon. I wanted to hear him say that he had missed something when

I last saw him at the hospital and he now had all the answers with the new MRI results but that didn't happen. There wasn't any notable change between the two reports. It was more of the same old thing. Sorry, it's a shame but I have no answers for you. Have a nice life.

As I left his office, I had such despair. It had been foolish to pin all my hopes on him. I am human though and that is what I had done. Now here I was, broken.

* My family doctor is an extremely private person. I am proud and thankful to have him as my physician. Although he plays a pivotal role in my story, I shall honour his privacy by changing his name to Dr. Welsh.

The Prescription Fix

Drug store medications like Tylenol didn't touch the pain. I tried so many pain medications that I can't honestly name them all. Dr. Welsh stopped prescribing me anything in any large quantity as they were a waste of time and money if they didn't do the trick. I would try something, wait and see how it worked, and then move on to something else, in the hopes that I would find a fix. I wonder if that is how the word "fix" came to describe taking drugs. The addict was just trying to find something to "fix" the problem, just like I was doing.

As it turns out, no one medication would do it all. After many months of trial and error, we settled on a combination of three powerful drugs. One of the drugs was a narcotic, while the other two were classed as anticonvulsants. One was for pain, and the other two were for something called break-out pain, the residual pain you get when the pain medications you are taking can't handle it all. Lord help me! Even taking those three medicines, my pain was acute. Where do you go, when you need break-out pain medication, for your break-out pain's break-out pain? It boggles the mind.

I simply wanted something that would take the edge off without making me feel heavy-headed and soulless. I would settle for things being manageable. I convinced myself that It didn't need to stop the pain entirely, some relief was better than none.

As each year passed, I was feeling more hollow inside. My pilot light was still functioning emotionally but at a reduced level. Instead of being an inferno, it resembled campfire embers by this point. My vitality and zest for life had gone into hiding.

When I was dealing with my knee injury, I had two very dangerous experiences with prescriptions that made me become extremely wary of drugs. I had had a really bad side effect on one of the medications and it entirely changed my personality. I got nasty, really nasty. I would snap at anyone, which was out of character because I was never known to have such a short fuse. I also had endless nausea. I was constantly bitchy, and nothing was ever good enough.

This was how bad it got. My poor Kim had done something super sweet for me for Christmas. He had gone to a fabric shop with a close friend of ours that was a seamstress. Together Kim and Sheila chose a simple pattern for me to make because I was a novice when it came to using a sewing machine. They had picked out material, a zipper, buttons, threads, interfacing, absolutely everything I could want in order to make myself an outfit. Not only was that an exceptionally thoughtful gift, but he had gone to the trouble to recruit Sheila to make certain that everything was perfect, not to mention this would have taken them both a lot of time and effort to pull off.

How did I thank him? I opened the gift up, took one look, and my exact words to him were, "What the hell do you expect me to do with this?" There wasn't a thank you sweetheart anywhere in sight. To this day, I try not to think about that moment because it makes me cringe. My actions were inexcusable. I never speak like that. I don't even think like that, never mind say such things. Yet on Christmas, of all days that was exactly what I said to him.

I stopped taking the medicine right away after that outburst. Two weeks later I read in the paper that the medication I had been taking was recalled because it was deemed unsafe, having led to the deaths of three people. That could have been me.

The second incident was only a month or so after the first. I had been given a prescription for a new medication and had it filled. I took it as prescribed and needed a repeat. When I collected the refill, it looked nothing like what I had been taking: not only was it a different colour, but a different shape as well.

I took the medication back to the pharmacist who insisted that this was the correct prescription. "It can't be," I protested. These aren't the same as the first pills given to me. Naturally, the pharmacy records had shown me getting the medicine that it says was prescribed the first time. I had no pills left to show them what I had taken, so there was no way to know what that mystery substance was. One of the prescriptions had clearly been wrong. What the hell had I put into my body? I never set foot inside that store again.

The universe was trying to tell me something. These two events changed my outlook on prescriptions. When it comes to medication, I always want to be a minimalist. It was an internal tug of war once the neurological pain got out of control. As much as I was against it, it had become a matter of necessity. I had fought a good fight, but resistance was futile.

Talk about a descent. I was in free-fall and heading for a mighty crash landing. I didn't dare try and add any other drugs. If I had been a dog or a cat, someone would have taken pity on me and put me out of my misery.

At my worst, I was seeing my family doctor every single week. I was a mess and getting worse with each passing day. How had I gotten into such a predicament? I was now nothing more than a walking, medicated zombie.

The narcotic that the doctor and I reluctantly agreed upon was methadone. I don't know what I was expecting, but I was surprised when it came in liquid form. It seemed more dangerous to me in liquid form rather than just another pill to take. I had a choice of cherry or orange flavour. The first time I filled the prescription it came in orange, so I just continued with that. I was given some small syringes to take home so that I could measure the exact dose. I got several because over time the ink would rub off of the syringe and I couldn't tell where the fill mark was.

I was so thankful that it didn't involve needles. I am fine about getting blood drawn, but giving a needle to myself was something entirely different. Oral ingestion at home was much easier. I just had to measure out the required dose and either squirt it into my mouth or, as I came to prefer, put it in a drop of orange juice and drink it.

I never let Kim measure out my methadone medication for me. Not because he wasn't competent enough; he could have and was willing to. I explained to him that it was important to me that I be the one to measure the methadone out. If I made a mistake and it killed me, I would be the one at fault—he wouldn't have to live the rest of his life blaming himself for accidentally causing my death. If he misread the syringe or somehow gave me too much, he wouldn't be able to live with himself. I would hate for him to go through that.

Right from the very beginning, I was in charge of anything to do with methadone. I had some tiny glass cups and would measure out the doses I needed for the day and place them safely in a separate compartment of the refrigerator door. Once they were in the fridge, I could get one or Kim could just grab one and bring it to me when I needed it.

I felt a sense of dread the first time that I took methadone. I was really petrified and had a cold sweat. I stood there for the longest time, trying to convince myself that I could just live with the pain. It wasn't too late, I could just walk away. I knew that once I took the methadone, there was no turning back.

It's peculiar now that I think about it, but in the back of my mind I never consciously thought the pain would go away. It was my inner spark that wouldn't allow me to give up on the vision of being pain-free. I didn't have a sense that being on the methadone would be temporary. I think that was why I was shaking. I knew that this was a defining moment.

That's for proper drug users I told myself, that isn't who I am. How had things gotten to this point why am a standing in front of a narcotic prescription with my name on it and a syringe in my hand?

I had an arduous battle raging within me. The likes of which I had never experienced until this very moment. My rational side was screaming NO DON'T DO IT! For God's sake, come to your senses, be sensible, walk away while you can. While my emotional side was imploring me to stop the pain and endless suffering. I didn't know how much longer I could carry on, living on hope and nothing more. My pilot light wasn't feeling particularly strong that day.

Either way, I felt that I was letting myself down. If the emotional side of me won, I was sentencing myself to medicated numbness. Would this be the last moment that I would be capable of clear thought? Maybe it's already too late for that? If the rational side of me won, I would be in torture for the rest of my life. Can I live with that forever? Do I have that much internal strength?

I shut my eyes, ignored the internal screams, and consumed the methadone. Now what? I had no idea what it would do to me and waited apprehensively for the drug to take effect. Having nothing to compare it to, I had no way of knowing if it was going to make me see things, or alter how I thought. This had to be having an effect on the brain. What if it damaged it more? After all, isn't it my brain causing the problem? I was an emotional wreck.

I tried to keep my mind occupied, but it was impossible. All I could think about was, once it takes effect, is it going to make a difference? Can I please be pain-free? It did take the edge off of the pain, however, it was far from a wonder drug. For the most part, although the pain was still there, the shocks that left me screaming were less frequent. I was thankful for that. It was all a bit of an emotional letdown. I had naturally hoped it would be the answer to everything, and it wasn't.

It had taken years to find medication that helped me even a little. Although this wasn't even close to perfect, Dr. Welsh and I decided that unless a new drug became available, this was likely as good as we were going to get. Over time we changed doses depending on how I was doing, but I stayed with those three medications.

Methadone made me feel hollow and numb. I was existing, that was about it. It was its own form of life support I suppose. It was like being put into limbo until some cure could be found for my condition. Once found, I would be resuscitated cured, and could carry on living. That is all well and good except for the fact that the world doesn't stand still to give you a chance to get your life in order. While I was busy trying to put myself together time was marching on, hundreds of daily neurological zaps were leaving their mark on me emotionally and physically.

I knew that methadone was in my system, but it was always an intruder, lurking about at will. I never got past hating myself for taking it. Each dose of methadone made me feel like an absolute failure. I could smell my defeat. To me, it was always my fault that I was taking narcotics because it boiled down to me not taking good enough care of my body and putting myself in this situation. My body clearly shouldn't have me in charge.

This is of course ridiculous mental rubbish. I hadn't neglected or abused myself. Yet each and every time, the blame game played in my head as methadone slid past my lips.

I could hear my pilot light reminding me that this isn't how my story is supposed to end. I can't give up. This was no time to settle. I needed to dust myself off and go out there and find a cure no matter how many more people I had to see, or how many more tests I had to endure. Somewhere out there was the life I wanted. I just had to go out and find it.

What Have I Got Myself Into?

My life was going in the wrong direction and picking up momentum at an alarming pace. I was in freefall down a very black hole. It was a matter of debate whether I would live long enough to collect my old age pension. Although I spent most of my time there, our home was looking more like a hospital wing rather than a pleasant place to live.

Not only that, it didn't take long to discover that there was an unexpected consequence to being on methadone that no one prepared me for. Keep in mind that I was not on methadone for any drug dependency issue, only to control my relentless pain. If I was one of those rare individuals who happens to enjoy pain, I would have been having the time of my life. Sadly, like most of us, I do not love pain.

In order to be on the medication, I had to sign a care agreement with my doctor that gave him far-reaching powers over my life. He could (and did) request random drug tests by the method of his choice, even including obtaining a hair follicle if he deemed it was necessary. It was potentially providing the hair follicle that bothered me most, strangely enough. I was not a criminal. You can't demand a hair follicle from just anyone. I don't know the justice system, but I am pretty sure that you can't even obtain a hair follicle from a convicted criminal without some sort of court order.

I was limited to using only one pharmacy. The small win for me was I could choose which pharmacy. Once I had made that choice, however, I couldn't change it later on unless I had my doctor's approval to do so. It didn't matter if it was more convenient to pick up a prescription somewhere else on occasion. I had to go to my designated pharmacy. There were so many rules.

I can understand that people who were on methadone due to drug dependency had a higher probability of seeing multiple doctors or pharmacy-hopping to get what they wanted. That was obviously the clientele they were accustomed to dealing with, so that's why the restrictions were put in place. I was now being considered just another druggie. There should have been some way to evaluate an individual's risk of abusing the system before clamping down on everyone. As that wasn't possible, I had to follow the rules.

According to the agreement I wasn't allowed to drink alcohol either. I get that combining alcohol and prescription medications is never a wise move, however, having that choice taken from me was just another way that I was slowly losing myself. To say that I am a social drinker would be generous. I can enjoy a nice alcoholic beverage on occasion, I just never seem to think about it. So why was I making such a big freaking deal about it? It should have been something that I just took in stride, right? I surprised myself because it really annoyed me that I couldn't have a drink if I felt like it, common sense be damned.

The only thing that I could put this over-the-top reaction down to was, that I was realizing I had gotten past my best before date. I was beyond fed up of restrictions. It's time to take your meds, Maria. You can't get your prescription here, Maria. Did you ask your doctor if it's okay, Maria? You mustn't have a drink, Maria. I was in medical prison, and it was beginning to look like I had been jailed for life.

The last thing I wanted to do was to sign that agreement. I was told that the choice is entirely mine to sign or not, but when it comes right down to it, I didn't get a choice. I was wedged between a rock and a hard place. I had declined to such a level that I agreed to things that I would never have considered before. If I failed to follow the rules my doctor could simply withhold his care until I complied.

Where I live, we have a critical shortage of physicians. There are honestly thousands of people who don't have a family doctor, so the thought of having a good doctor and not being able to see him was frightful. When you have complex medical concerns, you avoid a walk-in clinic whenever possible. Even Dr. Welsh told me not to go to a walk-in clinic unless his office was closed and it was something ordinary like suspected bronchitis. If it was anything serious, then his instructions were to avoid the clinic and go straight to the emergency department. I held on to the papers for several days before caving in and signing on the bottom line.

Dr. Welsh and I did negotiate that on special occasions I could have a drink, but for my own good, it should be only one glass. I was smiling on the inside because he never said what size the glass had to be. I wasn't going to be stupid and ask for clarification on the point. I was simply playing mental games, I knew what he meant but enjoyed a brief moment when I had discovered a loophole. As far as alcohol was concerned my social drinking fit well within his parameters of acceptable behaviour.

I had allowed myself to be tormented by the whole thing, making it a bigger deal than perhaps it should have been. Over time, when you are in a state of constant fight or flight, you just get worn down and even seemingly minor things can put you on edge. You are so used to fighting in one form or another that you lose the ability to let go of the simple things anymore. Is it any wonder then, why I had become so battle-weary? The paperwork was placed into my file and we never spoke about it again.

It isn't as though my doctor was picking on me because I was on methadone now. He was regulated by the government to get me to sign the agreement and to perform routine drug testing. The situation was out of our hands.

I will always remember the first time that I went for a random drug test. I was so naive. I went to the reception area with the requisition in my hand. It was a lab that I had used many times before. Although they were always polite and professional there, this time it felt judgmental. To be honest, every time after that when I was subjected to the test, I felt that I was being judged. In reality, they probably didn't give the encounter another thought, my brain couldn't see it that way though. It was as though all eyes were on me, and any quiet conversations the employees were having among themselves were about me. I would tell myself to get over it, that they weren't talking about me. The thing is, sometimes I don't listen to myself.

I was given a container to use to provide my sample, but was told that I was not allowed to take my purse or coat with me. If I had pockets, they had to be be empty. I was confused. Oh my God, I thought, were they concerned that I had a urine sample tucked into my purse, and that I was just waiting for the opportunity to switch it out when no one was looking? I might have used my coat pockets to conceal something, too, I suppose. Where the hell is my regular, nice private life? Fortunately, Kim went with me that day, so I was able to leave my purse and coat with him.

Whenever I am at a lab, I wash my hands before using the toilet, and then again afterward. I turned the tap on and there was no water. I went back to the receptionist and told her that there was something wrong with the bathroom sink, as the water wasn't working.

"Oh!" she said, "You aren't allowed water."

I beg your pardon, what do you mean? I thought. Do you actually expect me to go to the bathroom without washing my hands? I was trying, with every fibre of my being, not to burst into tears on the spot. The situation was barbaric. I returned to the bathroom as quickly as possible. I didn't want Kim to see me distressed, and just wanted to get this whole nightmare over and done with.

Once I provided the sample, I couldn't just hand it in and go. I had to wait while they tested it for the presence of illegal drugs. What were they going to do if they found something, call the police and have me arrested? They probably would have. I knew that they weren't going to find anything unexpected. That didn't stop me from wanting to dart toward the closest exit and make my escape. Once I was given the all-clear, the water was turned back on and I could clean myself up, gather my things and leave. I asked Kim if he thought I was being a drama queen letting myself feel traumatized like that. He said that he didn't know, all he could say was that he was glad it wasn't him. I had freely signed the consent form, now I had to accept that there would be many more random drug tests in my future. Hopefully, now that I know what to expect, things will get easier.

Each time after that, when I saw Dr. Welsh and hadn't been tested recently, I found myself making sure I wore a coat that wouldn't upset me if it had gotten stolen. I would have wet wipes with me to use upon arrival and only bring along essentials. If I could get away without taking a purse, I was even happier.

I didn't have a choice, if my doctor asked for a test, I couldn't say no to him. I couldn't tell him that I would rather have the test another day because I had a purse with me or had a drink the night before. That's not how it works. If he wanted a test done, I did it. I soon got a sense of how frequent the tests would be, which helped immensely. There is something unnatural about continually proving you are playing by all of the rules when you aren't giving anyone a reason to believe you are cheating.

Of course, there are people required to do random drug testing for a variety of reasons. They could be a commercial bus driver required by law to be screened for public safety purposes, or an athlete training for an international event. Perhaps their experience differed from mine. The most common reason, though, had to be because of drug addiction issues. It didn't matter what had brought us all here, we all found ourselves in the same boat, sitting at the lab waiting to be tested without water or coats, and nothing but empty pockets.

Although I didn't owe anyone an explanation, I found myself almost begging to make things clear and explain that it was all due to pain management and nothing more. Why the opinion of anyone else mattered to me about such things is something I can't explain. The more I tried to shake things off, the more it mattered.

If I could offer a word of advice to everyone who deals with people with chronic issues it would be this: don't let yourself see them as anything other than the people that they are. There are as many different reasons why people are in their current condition as there are health concerns generally. It doesn't really matter how they got where they are—either poor lifestyle choice, genetics, accident, or just some random twist of fate—we are all people.

In Dr. Welsh's defence, he was quite sweet, really. Knowing that he had no choice but to do the random drug testing, he would often try and lighten the mood. Once, I clearly remember around Christmas time, he joked that with the holiday cocaine party scene just around the corner, he thought we should get the drug test done and out of the way before the festivities really got rolling. He knew me well by this point and understood my sense of humour. He recognized the only reason he was asking wasn't to find any illegal substance. It was a legislated requirement that we both had to follow, that was all, and we were in this together. We both chuckled as I grabbed the requisition from his hand and made my way down the hall to the lab.

Giving Up Was Becoming a Possibility

Of all my medications, the methadone was the most crucial to keep on a rigid schedule: 5 a.m., 1 p.m., 9 p.m., sleep and repeat, day in and day out, year in and year out. If we were out longer than anticipated and I didn't have the methadone with me at medication time, we had to go back home so that I could take it, no questions asked. Nothing was more important than my next dose. The drugs controlled me, they held the key to any kind of relief. Medication was a necessary evil in my world, part friend, part sworn enemy. Dr. Welsh assured me that I was drug dependent not drug-addicted, there was a subtle difference in the wording I'll give him that. Would I get to the point where my dependence became an addiction? Only time would tell.

Once we were home and the medication took effect, we never went back out again. I didn't have the stamina to continue. Whatever we had planned to do was scrapped. We were going to be in now for the rest of the day. I might as well get changed, put my slippers on, and head back to the couch. There I would be until my last medication and bedtime.

I don't know why I bothered to refer to it as bedtime. Yes, I was physically in a bed, but you couldn't really tell the difference between my awake time and my sleeping time. I was either in bed or on the couch. Either way, I was horizontal for a large part of the day. The only difference was that I was doing it in two different rooms, that's all.

The methadone needed to be kept cold, which presented its own set of logistical nightmares. Trying to actually experience life while maintaining the medicine schedule was taxing. Things got a bit better once I found cooling pouches that are used by diabetics to keep insulin cold. It was a small cloth pouch with an inner section that you could pull out. All you had to do was put this inner section into cold water. There was something in there that made it swell up but the cold would stay for hours. By placing the methadone inside the pouch my medication was able to stay at a suitable temperature whenever I was away from home. That was a game-changer for me.

The next time I was at the drug store I asked for a couple of their smallest medicine bottles. By this time, I was a very familiar face to them, so they were happy to give them to me. From that point on, when I was out and needed to keep the methadone cool, I simply took one of my pre-measured doses from the refrigerator, poured it into the medicine bottle, and into the sack. It worked really well.

There was a lot of trial and error back in the early days, as Kim and I navigated this new reality. We found a way to make it all work. It would have been so much easier if someone had handed us a cheat sheet, that's for sure.

There were major restrictions regarding methadone over

and above the agreement I signed. I was one of the fortunate ones, if you could call it that. Because I was on methadone for pain relief, I did not have to go down daily to the pharmacy and have them administer it for me. I was spared the humiliation of being watched to make certain I had consumed it. I was allowed a 45-day supply, but no more. I was trusted to administer it at the required times and in the correct dose. In that sense, the powers that be did at least let me try and get on with things.

I could not even request a repeat prescription until the day before it was due. So no matter what I was doing on the 45th day, I better get my ass down to the only pharmacy I had agreed to use and get the prescription. If it was a particularly bad day for me pain-wise, they would allow Kim to pick the methadone up on my behalf. He was the only other person that was allowed to do that for me, and I had to let the pharmacy know ahead of time if that was going to happen. We also had to always sign that we had received the prescription. It was a government requirement and they kept really tight controls.

There was one time this restriction really hit home for me. Because my hands were very shaky and holding the bottle made my hand hurt, I actually spilled some methadone, equal to several days' supply. I was devastated. It hadn't been just the single dose from the refrigerator door, I could have lived with that. This was a partially used bottle. I was frantically attempting to syringe the liquid back up, but my efforts were futile. There was no extra and no hope of getting any. I was screwed.

My only option was to take a smaller dose each time until I had made up for what I had spilled. You aren't supposed to tamper with your medicine levels, however, what choice did I have? I had to make up for the day's worth of methadone laying in a small pool before me. I wouldn't be back to a full dose for more than a week. That really messes you up big time. I was about to experience the effects of opiate withdrawal. You would think that a little less medicine shouldn't be a problem. My body noticed quickly and was waging war on me in protest.

I had to find just the right balance between keeping my pain level tolerable and getting back to a proper dose as soon as I could. I cut back just enough that I felt the difference, but didn't get violently sick. It was a few rough days, but my method managed to limit the damage.

I really needed to pay extra attention now that my hands were hurting more, whenever I was dealing with methadone. I wasn't quite ready to hand over methadone responsibility to Kim, but if it happened again, it might be my only option.

This was something more I had to watch out for. Life was getting more difficult by the day. I was relying heavily on my pilot light. Each challenge made it harder to imagine a life of health and fun.

When exactly was I going to say enough is enough? If restrictions weren't doing it, all the drugs weren't doing it, is there anything that could shake me up enough to change a single thing about how I was living? Any common sense on the matter was long gone. I wasn't even playing an active role in finding solutions anymore. I was all wrapped up in existing, rather than living.

Whenever I was solely in self-survival mode, I had to hope that my pilot light was on the autopilot setting. I wasn't giving it much attention when actually it should have been my priority. There were too many things demanding my attention simultaneously, that in my medicated state it somehow made sense to let my spark take care of itself. It was during those misguided times that the possibility of giving up would cross my mind. Fortunately, my pilot light won't accept that. I always heard in the back of my mind that change was just another word for transition. It didn't automatically make something inherently bad or good. If things were not how I wanted them to be I needed to run toward change rather than from it. My pilot light was the fuel to enable a transformation to happen. I needed to have my pilot light action-ready at all times.

Although I am usually a very upbeat person, the years of living on a physical and emotional rollercoaster were taking a toll. Antidepressants had been offered, which I thought about, and eventually decided against. It was more important for me to know that I was having a good day because I was actually having a good day, than it was to take the medication. I appreciated the offer and knew I could ask for them if I ever changed my mind. I was on enough medication as it was. I wasn't moving hardly at all. Even though I ate very little, the pounds kept piling on each time I got on the scale. I wasn't mobile enough to lose any weight no matter how small my portions were. My solution was to stop getting on the scale. I was searching for new clothes every few weeks because I had already outgrown the ones that I had just bought.

One time I wanted to buy something nice to wear because we were going to Kim's staff Christmas party. I wasn't going for 'looking fabulous' because, in my mind, I was way beyond that possibility. I figured with some effort I could pull off feeling pretty.

It was a massive undertaking to go out looking for fancier clothes. Although Kim hates to shop unless it's for bicycle parts, he offered to take me anywhere I wanted to go. We made sure I had all the medicine I needed with us and started shopping at one of the larger malls, and then went to another one when I couldn't find anything. If I liked something it wasn't available in my size or what was available in my size was hideous and old-looking. The orthotics would have completed the outfit nicely.

We were getting to the end of a very difficult day and still hadn't found anything that I wanted to wear. I suggested that Kim go to the party alone, but he wouldn't hear of it. In a last-ditch effort, we ended up driving to a small community about 40 minutes away.

As we walked along their main road, we found a small ladies clothing shop. We went in and started to browse. At first, nothing grabbed my attention. I was feeling pretty desperate at this point, so decided to go through the store one more time before we wrote it off. I even had Kim willingly watch for anything he thought would be worth trying on. This shop was my last hope as time was running out.

Out of the corner of my eye, tucked off to the side, was not one but two pretty tops. One was sparkly and the other one had a shimmer that was really cool. It was copper, but depending on how the light was shining on it, it would change colour. I tried the copper one on and it looked lovely on me. It managed to make me feel pretty. I felt like Cinderella going to the ball.

I was ready to buy it when Kim suggested that I should try the black one on seeing as I had it right there in the change room with me. The sparkly black top looked pretty too, so he told me to take both. I have a hunch he was thinking that if I had a second nice top if another special occasion presented itself, he wouldn't have to go through the shopping ordeal again. He is a very smart man that way. Even if that was the reason behind him saying to take both, it was just like Kim to be so sweet. He didn't even look at the price tag, bless him. To him, my smile was priceless.

We had achieved success but outings like these always came at a price. The following day I was bedridden. I didn't even make it to the couch. The only time I left the bed was to go to the bathroom. We always had to allow for recovery time. We got to know what my estimated recovery time would be depending on the activity we were planning. But this time I was happy to go through the needed recovery period because I knew that come the following weekend I would feel pretty when I went out with Kim.

Thinking Outside the Box

When something truly horrible is happening to you, and it persists for years, it becomes almost impossible not to regress into your own world. When there were other people around, I put on a good show, but when I was alone with my thoughts it was really easy to see the reality I was living with and what my future was potentially going to look like. I might not have wanted to acknowledge what was going on with me physically, but I was acutely aware that I was in a bad way and getting worse.

It became almost a panic, because the longer it continued the worse it was going to be. I would lay awake thinking, "If this is bad, what will next week, or next month look like?" The deeper I sank into the hole, the harder it would be to escape. My pilot light would have moments of brightness, but for the most part, it was bloody hard work to remain upbeat. These weren't mood swings; when my light would flicker it was because I was weary from fighting. I needed rest, but there just wasn't any to be had.

The weekly appointment with Dr. Welsh was an arduous outing. It took a concerted effort to get there, but it reminded me that someone was on my side. On one of these visits, we decided that I should go and see the neurosurgeon that the professor had talked about. What did I have to lose?

When I saw the neurosurgeon four or five months later, I was emotionally numb. There wasn't the usual anticipation, I didn't care enough to be excited or hopeful. The internal screaming to get anyone to notice me had gone eerily quiet. My pilot light was flickering. I didn't have it in me to fan the flames that day.

Our meeting started with her saying that she wanted to perform a nerve conduction test on me. I was immediately transported back to the ordeal with the physiatrist years before. Was that the only test there was? I wanted to say no, we're done, but the mind is a peculiar beast. I had waited so long to see her that I thought I had to let her do what she thought she needed to do, even if I didn't want it.

She was a petite Eastern European woman, and as I sat there, I thought of how much she would have had to go through to get where she was professionally. Neurosurgeons are at the top of the heap when it comes to medical specialties. There she was, a woman in a male-dominated field, highly educated, and speaking to me in complex medical terms in a language that was clearly not her mother tongue. This was an amazingly smart woman, why would I get in the way of hearing what she had to say?

The nerve conduction test was every bit as painful as I had remembered it. It might have been even harder to get a successful test conducted because I knew what to expect. I was tensing up the moment I was advised that it was about to start. No amount of telling myself to take a deep breath and relax did a blind bit of good. Even parts of me that weren't normally tense were getting into the act.

I asked her why the problems had started just out of the blue that day when I experienced my first jolt of pain. She went into great detail about thinking of the brain as being divided into a bunch of drawers or boxes. When your brain can't do something the usual way, it tries to use another drawer instead. Eventually, though all the drawers get filled and your brain can't perform the function. I took that as just another way of saying that she was now on the ever-growing list of people who couldn't help me.

I was shocked the next time that I went for my regular doctor appointment when I was told that the neurosurgeon had recommended that I have a muscle biopsy done to explore the possibility that I might have corrupted DNA. She hadn't said a word to me about it when I met her in person. It annoyed me that something that sounded pretty serious to me didn't even rate a mention. Maybe she is old-school and talks only with other doctors, who knows. Perhaps collectively everyone was running out of ideas to help me and this was some last-ditch effort on her part in order to come up with a cause or cure.

How on earth would a person get corrupted DNA, I asked myself. If they find out I have corrupted DNA, what can they do for me? Can they fix it? What would fixing it entail? Something that sounded horrible would likely have just as horrible a solution. I had a million and one questions running through my head.

In Dr. Welsh's calming manner, he advised me not to get ahead of myself. I was to think of it as just another test and a great opportunity to rule something sinister out of the equation. That made sense, but we are talking about a possible problem with my DNA and not some blood test or urine sample.

The muscle biopsy couldn't be done in the town where I live. There was only one place in the province where I could have the procedure performed and it would be an all-day adventure to get there.

Arranging the logistics of getting there and back put me in a bit of a tailspin. The provincial medical plan did give me a voucher to help with a portion of my travel expenses, but all of the pieces had to come together just right in order to pull this off.

Because my medication would make me nod off almost without warning, I hadn't driven in years. I thought about taking buses, but that would have involved many bus changes. I would be going to a much bigger city and I wouldn't have a clue how to get where I needed to go. One wrong move and I would be hooped. If the appointment was too early, we would have to travel there the day before, and if it was too late, Kim couldn't drive me because he can only drive in daylight.

Whatever appointment I got I had to take. I told my friend Judy about the appointment, simply bringing her up to date, when she offered to take me.

I fought back tears when I asked her if she really meant that. She said, "Of course I do, or I wouldn't have said it." I reminded her that she would be dealing with a lot of traffic because it was in the city, but that didn't dissuade her. What a remarkable generous woman. I don't know many people that would do that without a great deal of persuasion.

The appointment was arranged through the neurosurgeon's office. Like all specialist appointments, it took months to come through. Because I was getting physically weaker the longer my nightmare continued, I was now using a walker whenever I went outside of the house. On the designated day, Judy and I loaded up the walker and took off. The journey itself was quite pleasant. We had managed to get something nice to eat and had lots of time for a great chat. The time had passed by far quicker than I had anticipated.

The procedure was being performed in what I would call the medical district. It was in a very busy part of town and although it was connected to the hospital, it was a couple of city blocks away from the main hospital building itself. All along the street were similar structures of four or five storeys, each of them pertaining to a different area of expertise and all of them part of the hospital. It reminded me of being on a university campus. It had its own identity. It felt like a small city within a city. Parking prices were prohibitive, if I remember correctly it was $20 for the first 90 minutes, then $10 an hour after that. Highway robbery it may have been, but as there was no street parking you were given no choice but to pay.

The building was state of the art. It had a very large concourse area with various rooms along each side. It wasn't just one department like I thought it would be. There were all sorts of different procedures taking place.

Our appointment was fairly late in the day, so by then, the appointments were running late. We easily waited 90 minutes to be seen, even though the procedure wasn't supposed to take more than a few minutes. It was just as well that we were not parked on a meter or our time would have already been up. Unfortunately, when it got to my turn, the person conducting the procedure couldn't locate the muscle she was looking for in order to take my sample.

I had not contemplated that finding a muscle would be hard. It just makes sense, though, when you think about it: I had been sedentary for years, obviously my muscles had atrophied. I don't know if she was a doctor or a technician, but she was almost at the point of giving up. There was nothing for pain, probably because the procedure is usually quick and easy, making medication unnecessary.

The muscle she wanted was from my left thigh. She was on a mission, and began diving deeply into my flesh. At first, the pain was tolerable, but once it went beyond a muscle search to a gouging operation, everything changed. It really hurt. To my relief, she got the sample she had been searching for, and then, she made a point saying that she had never had a muscle biopsy that was so challenging to do. I have a small permanent scar on my left thigh as a souvenir from my experience.

By the time we were done, I was done in. I was so happy to get that over with. I thought that the testing to see if I had corrupted DNA was going to be done in Canada. I was wrong, in actual fact, the only place that was doing this specific test was at the Centre for Disease Control in Atlanta.

Imagine my surprise when, as I was about to leave, I was given a form to fill out which turned out to be a passport application for my DNA. Obviously, it looked slightly different than a personal passport form, but it was official paperwork to allow my DNA to enter America. I found the thought of it really hysterical and was having a hard time containing my laughter. In my head I was picturing the very serious-looking photos that you need to have taken when applying for a passport, and whether someone had to take a photo of the specimen they had collected for identification purposes. The absurdity of it all really set me off. It was the best laugh I had had in a very long time.

The results took several months to come back. I was relieved to discover that there was nothing sinister to report. That was a weight off of my shoulders because I was quite confident that if it had been anything bad, there wouldn't be anything that could be done about it. It was probably going to result in my early death.

Answers Change Depending on Who is Asking

After the DNA exploration had not proven helpful, I was back to only the routine weekly visits to Dr. Welsh. I must have been seven or eight years into the ordeal, maybe longer. Time had become a blur. Everything had a sense of hurry-up-and-wait about it. After each specialist appointment, Dr. Welsh would explain to me in words that I could understand what they had written in their assessment report.

We had explored every avenue possible by this point, or so I thought. Just when I believed I had reached the end of my road, Dr. Welsh decided to try and get me in to see a neurological physiotherapist. They deal with a lot of stroke patients and people with traumatic brain injuries. Mine wasn't a traumatic injury, but clearly, my brain had a defect, whether I was born with it or my drawers were full my brain had issues.

I had never known that these types of specialists existed. My referral was sent in, along with my pertinent medical history. It was a six-week program that was paid for by my local health system. Patients who were accepted into the program met with a neurological physiotherapist twice a week for an hour. If they saw good progress, they had the option of extending my enrolment to twelve weeks, but that was the maximum allowed no matter how you were doing. I did explore the possibility of paying privately should things be going well, but was told that was not an option.

For the first time since the professor left town, I felt a glimmer of hope. I eagerly went for the assessment. It was supposed to take a minimum of an hour, but it was over almost before it had started. The assessor took one look at me, asked me a couple of questions, and on the spot declared that I didn't qualify for the program. I was there for less than 15 minutes.

Case closed, it was just another colossal waste of time and effort.

On the next visit to Dr. Welsh, he told me that he had tried to contact the neurosurgeon multiple times. She had failed to return his messages. He rarely passed any judgment, but did say it was a matter of professional courtesy that she should at the very least return his calls.

Obviously, at some point, they must have had a conversation, because I was notified by my doctor's receptionist a week or two later that an appointment had been made for me to see the people running the neurological physiotherapy department. I wasn't hopeful. I had just been down that road.

When I got there for my second attempt, things were very different. I was asked the same questions as before. My answers had not changed, nor had my medical history, the only difference was that the referral came from a neurosurgeon rather than a family physician.

I expected to hear "no" the entire way through the process.

They were much more thorough the second time. I wasn't being dismissed. There was great attention to detail and personal engagement from the staff. For once, I left victorious. I had been accepted into the program and it would start in three weeks. I was elated.

If Dr. Welsh had not gone to bat for me, I wouldn't have had the opportunity to do this. I was not going to waste a single moment. I was going to give it everything I had. I was going to get them to extend the program to twelve weeks come hell or high water. Those next few weeks felt like waiting for Christmas to come.

There was a mix of excitement and nervousness when the day arrived for me to start the program.

There wasn't a bunch of fancy equipment. There were two recumbent exercise bikes, and what looked like everyday things you would find at home. A ball here, some straps there. It didn't look glitzy like so many other hospital departments. It was plain, but totally functional. They had everything they needed, it just wasn't filled with medical paraphernalia which surprised me.

A lovely lady by the name of Pam was my therapist. It takes a tremendous amount of education in order to become a neurological physiotherapist, so there was absolutely no doubt that I was in the hands of a very smart woman. She was young and bubbly, very dedicated to her profession. She meant business when it came to getting down to the task at hand, but I was still allowed to have some fun, as long as I remained active the entire time we were together.

The first appointment was a series of tests, things like sitting on a chair, but I had to try to get up without using the arms for support. The same thing applied to sitting down: could I do it without needing help. I won't go into details of each test as it was just an assessment. I failed almost all of them, and those I did manage to pass, it wasn't with a high grade.

I never saw more than a couple of extra clients at the clinic, it was very private. Over the weeks I would see others doing new things and marvel at how far they had come. The same was true for me. Pam used a lot of resistance bands and weighted balls. I would stand in a corner so that I wouldn't fall over and then Pam would pass me a ball, have me shut my eyes, bend my knees and try to make a quarter-turn stand up straight and open my eyes. Because I was so unstable on my feet, this exercise was exceptionally hard to do. All of the sessions were rapid-fire. I wasn't given time to think. We went from one exercise to the next, then immediately onto the next thing. The longest time I spent on any one task was 20 minutes on the exercise bike which was the very first thing that we would do when I arrived. The rest of the time we would switch what we were doing every few minutes.

One particular day close to the six-week mark, Pam had put me on a mini trampoline which she had placed safely between two balance bars. We then tried to do the same exercise I had been doing in the corner with my eyes shut and the quarter turn. It didn't look pretty; every move took my total concentration. I did it though, without falling off.

When I came home, I was bursting to tell Kim that I had been on a mini-trampoline.

"No, you didn't," he insisted.

"I did, I did, you should have seen me," I gushed.

Neurological physiotherapy worked. When the six-week mark came, I anxiously waited to hear if my time would be extended. I had worked incredibly hard and was praying that I had done enough to impress Pam into letting me stay longer. It wasn't until we were finished our session that she told me I could have another six weeks. Hallelujah! I had made it, let the celebration begin. I was ecstatic.

Pam told me that the reason they don't just automatically make the program twelve weeks for everyone was that a lot of people don't put in the effort. Because this was such a specialized program, they didn't want to tie up a place with someone who wasn't going to gain anything. This way, they tried it for a few weeks to see what the client would do, what effort they were willing to put in, then it was up to the therapist to decide if they were going to invest more time and effort into training. This also allowed more access to the program for more people. As soon as someone dropped out at the six-week mark or graduated after twelve, there was another patient given the opportunity to benefit from the program.

At the end of the twelve weeks, I did all of my original tests again, but instead of failing, I aced them all, plus a few new ones. Somewhere buried in a memorabilia box, I still have the "report card" she had given me showing that I had gotten all A's.

We were both congratulated by Pam's colleagues which I thought was very sweet. It was nice that they had noticed our efforts. Not everyone's journey has the same happy ending as I had. I couldn't help but think that this opportunity could have very easily slipped through my fingers were it not for Dr. Welsh getting the neurosurgeon to submit my name.

With all my progress, I had not considered that what goes up has to come down. In hindsight, I wish I had given it some thought. I was so pleased with myself, and rightly so. It was the first positive thing to happen to me health-wise in probably close to a decade. When my program ended, it was almost inevitable that I would crash down to earth at some point. My pain levels hadn't altered, but I had a brand-new feeling of freedom and mobility at first. What I had not mentally prepared myself for was that once it was over, it was truly over. It was as though it had all been a dream. I couldn't contact Pam or the department once I had left, you needed to be a current client for that. There was no referral to anyone who provided neurological physiotherapy in the community. I couldn't find anyone that did what Pam could do, even though I tried. I was annoyed. How unfair is that: I proved that I was getting somewhere. by following what I had learned. How can they expect that to continue without any kind of follow-up? I looked great on paper; my results were through the roof. Somewhere in the medical system, I was a triumphant success story. Job well done. Now they moved onto the next person in the system while I was abandoned. Even with my best efforts, it was just a matter of months before I was back to how things were. I was actually worse off, at least mentally speaking. I had had a very small taste of how things could be, and now it was gone. Instead of being happy-go-lucky or thankful, I was resentful. I wanted to keep going. I had finally, after all these years, found something that was improving my quality of life. No sooner had I found it, it was taken away again. It was a sick joke, and I felt more hopeless than ever.

The Difficulties of Daily Life

My time with Pam had been my only ray of light in otherwise endless darkness. After the sessions ended, I made every effort to keep up with what I had learned; however, things soon returned to their downward trajectory. This was much harder to accept now that I had proof that certain things could be a lot better than they were.

Waking from my medicated slumber each morning, it would take a few minutes to realize that it was a new day. In my world, the only difference from one day to the next was what I might find to watch on the television.

I didn't know what day it was, and frankly, I didn't care. All I cared about was when was I going to get the next dose of drugs to numb the pain. The medication wouldn't take away the pain entirely, instead, I just settled for a scrap of relief. My life had become all about settling.

As I laid in bed trying to get my bearings, I would feel that familiar formation taking place. It would start off small at first, a tightness running down my leg usually from my knee past the tip of my toes right to the very end of my toenails. The tightness would intensify; my body knew what was coming, but was powerless to prevent it. When it was at its peak, I got an overwhelming electrical impulse, a charge that ran right along my nerves. It is how I imagine a jolt from a taser would feel. They were so intense, even though I knew what was coming, they still managed to steal my breath away. Try as I might to remain silent, I would cry out in pain when the severity got more than I could bear.

I was thankful to have survived. I would take a recovery breath in, only to realize that the formation had already begun again. This was a repeating cycle with only the very briefest of breaks between them from the moment I woke until I went to sleep at night.

I would reach over to find the medication that I needed on the nightstand. Kim would make certain it was there each morning like clockwork. My life was so structured around medication and finding relief. With the pills taken and the narcotic mixture drunk, I would lay back down and wait for the medicine to take effect.

Once the medication kicked in, was I suddenly ready to take on the day? Sadly no, I was nowhere near being full of life. The fact that I was still breathing was a win in my world. I would stay in bed a good part of the day lying there, watching my body tense and release. I would go to the kitchen for food only when I was so hungry that it was worth making the effort to get up and go a few feet to the kitchen.

I would try and rally my energy when I knew it was close to the time that Kim would be coming home from work. Who was I kidding? He knew things were bad, but in my medicated haze I thought that I could put on some sort of Oscar-worthy performance and convince him that I was fine.

Those attempts to look fine were exhausting. He was doing the same thing: he tried to remain strong enough for both of us and look after me, but the woman that he fell in love with and married showed little resemblance to the woman before him now. He became my caregiver decades before anyone is usually expected to be put in that position. He hadn't prepared himself for the reality we were both living, any more than I did, yet here we were.

I had become a medicated zombie unable to sustain any kind of normal life. The days of getting out in the car and having an adventure were long gone. The medicine would make me sleep. Without warning, I would be off in slumberland, which meant being behind a wheel wasn't an option. For the most part, I didn't mind the sleep, solely because it passed the time. Time became monotonous nothingness. The freedom to live life on my own terms was gone.

When I would make the extraordinary effort to actually leave the house there was always a price to pay. The medication would become less effective, while the nerve pain got stronger, and my recovery time was longer.

I didn't want to die, but no one would call this living. I was firmly in middle earth between living and dying, in my own form of solitary confinement. Something had to be done, yet all I was thinking was just give me the drugs and leave me on the couch. I'm done.

As things continued to take a downward slide, it became increasingly more difficult to hold onto anything in my hands. Kettles full of boiling water were not exactly good things for me to be lifting up. The hands become incredibly weak.

That happened lightning quick. Gone were the days where I could lift a saucepan or unscrew a lid, even with a device that was supposed to be able to open anything. It was a challenge to hold on to keys and unlock the door for heaven's sake. I would either drop the keys or fumble trying to figure out how to get the key into the lock. My life was going to hell.

My brain felt sticky, as though it had been covered by a thick layer of dust, everything took much more effort. My thoughts were no longer crystal clear or decisive, and my reaction time was extremely slow. I had been on the same group of medicines for a very long time and the cumulative effects were showing.

There were occasions where I would go to do something quite ordinary and not know how to get my body to do what I wanted it to do. It was as though my brain had deleted the file without my permission. I would need to use immense concentration to try and will myself to do something that had always been second nature to me.

I certainly couldn't retain anything new. Concentration was out of the question. The more that my brain felt sticky the more my neurological pains intensified. It was creating this perfect environment for my pain waves to run rampant.

My hair used to be lovely and thick, much more manageable than it is now. I was losing hair at an alarming rate. After having a bath and washing my hair, I would drain the water, only to discover a layer of hair left behind. Each time I would brush, I would gather up the hair and throw it away. The volume I once had was lost forever. Even my teeth began needing major work. I put it down to long-term prescription use. The drugs were going everywhere within my body and there was a price for that.

I didn't have a lot of energy; little things had become monumental challenges. Even stepping off of a curb had become next to impossible. I would literally stand there and not know how to get down. It's unbelievable to think things could get this bad, but they had. Often I would walk, shuffle along until I could find the slope that is at most of the busier corners and navigate my way down that way. Sometimes though there wasn't a slope, I had no choice but to somehow get myself down from the curb. There would be a hint of panic come over me. I would do one of three things:

I would lunge myself forward and pray that I didn't lose my balance entirely as I shakily attempted to lower myself down a few inches to safety.

If I had anything in my hands like a purse or shopping bags, I put them down on the sidewalk, and then got myself down by going backward, then pick my things up again, turn myself around and continue on once I had managed to restore what little balance I had.

Finally, if someone was going by and saw my ordeal, sometimes they would ask me if I was okay and offer to get me safely across the road.

As much as I always thought what a life-saver these people were, I would internally cringe that things had gotten to such an extreme. No wonder my family was concerned when I was out on my own. Someone should be with me anytime that I needed to leave the house, but that wasn't always possible. Sometimes I was in a scary world, and left to my own devices. I was a 90-year-old trapped in a body that was chronologically half that age.

I am surprised that I didn't develop full-on panic attacks about crossing the street when I was alone. Those timed crosswalks are never long enough. I would end up being in the middle of a busy intersection when they would run out of time. I didn't know whether to make my way back to the beginning and start again or say a prayer and continue to keep going.

These are the nightmares people with mobility issues face daily, and no one talks about it. It's okay for the able-bodied people who can strut across like they own the universe. If you aren't one of what the bureaucrats call an 'average member of society,' life can get pretty darn scary.

Escalators freak me out, especially those going down. When I am going up, a stair is formed which means I can't overstep and lose my balance. Going down often there is no visual indication of where my foot should be placed. There might be a line but they are going by so fast that I miss the visual aid. If I were to place my foot between steps, part of where I am standing moves when the stair is formed, and down I could potentially go.

I don't approach an escalator and simply get on, I freeze. I grab onto the handrail firmly and watch the escalator move to calculate the precise moment that I should step on to avoid falling. This always ends up in a misfire or two. By the time my brain says go, I have actually missed my opportunity and have to wait for the next step to appear.

I must seem very polite to people approaching, as I always offer to let them go ahead of me. I watch how they get on with ease and wonder how the hell they are doing that. I have better success if the escalator is on the slow side. Regardless of speed though, the procedure remains the same. If I have shopping bags with me, I avoid escalators.

My sister is with me quite often when I am out shopping. If she is there, she always asks me if I would prefer to use the elevator. If I decide to take the escalator, she grabs my purse and any shopping bags I have, so that all I need to do is get on. If we are going between floors and multiple escalators are involved, it gets too much to tackle so the elevator is my best option. I am always relieved when I successfully get on. There is a brief worry about stepping off, but it isn't as intense.

Going up or down regular stairs that do not have handrails is practically impossible as well. I have lost count of how many times I have faced that challenge. There have been plenty of places I couldn't go at all. I had to have something or someone to hold on to. If there were people sitting on the steps blocking the side with the handrail, I was going nowhere.

Even public arenas where I live don't have handrails all the way up the length of the bleachers for the spectators. If I was alone and someone offered to help me, I still had to think about how I was going to get back. Don't even get me started about any exit strategy should nature call.

One time, the Moody Blues were playing at the arena and Kim thought that it would be nice to go. Although it wasn't a band that sold out in the first two minutes, tickets were going fast. There were only two areas in the arena that I could navigate to my seat easily: the lower portion that had handrails or the very top row in a small area by the box seats. Kim did manage to get seats in the nosebleed section, and we had a lovely time. Because the seats were so limited though, and not always the best location to see what was going on, I never suggested going to see anything. It wasn't worth the effort, even if I would have enjoyed the act.

Sometimes even doing the things I loved was just too much effort. I become every bit as much of a weight lifter as the athletes lifting weights at the gym. You don't get any accolades though. No one says, "Well done, great job." You just find that you have no choice; you have to keep lifting.

Pain and my life, such as it was, had all the makings of a great action movie. There was the menacing attacker, the anguished victim, the rescue team of superheroes preparing to enter the danger zone. An epic fight to the death, no holds barred battle scene, intense drama and suspense, some heartache and loss, sprinkled with a bit of romance for good measure. Yes, I believe it had it all.

When you are in pain, you can't just get off of the couch and get on with things, it can feel as though you are fighting the overwhelming pull of earth's gravity single-handedly in order to achieve liftoff. It can take a Herculean effort to break free of the bonds that shackle us where we are. Some days my inner goddess just became battle weary.

I think that one of the biggest hurdles about living with chronic pain is that people can't see it. It is an invisible disability, and yet it is a disability in every sense of the word. It isn't as though there was a bandage, sling, or cast that alerted everyone around me that I was in pain, and please proceed with tender loving care.

I needed to develop an exceptionally high pain tolerance over the years. I might say that my pain level is at a five on a scale of 1–10, whereas someone else with the same pain level might call it a solid 10. If there was an Olympic event for pain tolerance, I would have easily made the national team and likely been on the podium. I was a professional after having years to perfect the craft.

Chronic illness is a heavyweight to carry and something that is always with you. There weren't days off, it was there for every single special occasion. It was present as I opened my Christmas and birthday gifts, year in and year out, just as it was an uninvited guest at weddings and any other special events we were invited to, even family reunions didn't constitute a reprieve. There was no on/off switch, and no one that I could leave my condition with while I went to have some fun.

Pain and chronic illness are life-altering not only for the individual, but for their family as well. It's the white elephant in the room that people would rather not acknowledge.

If You Can't Say Something Nice, Silence is Golden

Life changes when you become chronically ill. As if a serious medical condition wasn't enough to contend with. People started to see me as incapable. Yes, I was physically incapable of many things. It was the fact that people began to wrongly believe that I was mentally incapable as well that stung me the most. It was as though the only option to deal with me was to treat me like I was in my late nineties. I became someone to be tolerated. Just stick me in a corner and throw a blanket over me.

There are a lot of people who just don't come equipped with any sort of filter and find it perfectly acceptable to speak their mind when no one was soliciting their opinion.

Human nature is funny isn't it? The really bad things are etched into our memory and will remain with us forever. It seems to take countless good acts to compensate for just one bad thing. Even now, I am writing about the uncomfortable things I encountered, rather than the many acts of kindness bestowed upon me. Yet those kind acts meant the world to me.

I remember once being on holiday, we were shopping in a small town while waiting for our niece Erin to get off work. Someone stopped us, and as though I wasn't even there, said to Kim, that he had me looking nice today. What the heck? Kim just thanked her. What was he supposed to do with a comment like that?

To me, it felt like she was trying to acknowledge Kim's effort to look after me. Either that or she was digging hard to try and find something positive to say as she walked by rather than saying nothing. If a stranger says I look nice, it usually prompts a pleasant reaction, this time it was a backhanded compliment, and that's being generous. It implied to me that I couldn't look nice without having Kim's help.

Hands down the worse unprovoked personal attack I encountered was when I was spat on. For that, let me give you the back story.

Kim, an avid cyclist, had made valiant attempts to teach me how to ride over the years. Despite these efforts, I didn't have the balance required to ride a standard two-wheel bicycle. To get around my physical shortcomings we got a tandem. Kim put a great deal of effort into researching just the right manufacturer and model. Although my lack of balance created challenges for him, he managed to compensate as long as I didn't lean into the curves. He would joke that he considered me more as nice decorative luggage than he did as an assistant. I didn't take his assessment personally though. As long as I stayed still, he shifted his weight accordingly and we could ride. All I needed to do was hold on tightly and keep spinning. Over time I got good at spinning my legs. My extra horsepower helped when we were going up the hills and when it came to going downhill, we flew. We started to commute to work by bicycle and enjoyed it. I was finally able to share one of Kim's greatest passions.

Sadly, this was all before the demise of my health. As things went from bad to worse health-wise, I couldn't hold onto the handlebars tightly enough to hold on. Getting on and off the bike was no longer safe, so our days as tandem riders were behind us. We didn't go on a bike ride together for years after that.

One day out of the blue Kim began looking at trikes for me. He had never given up his dream of having a missus who could ride. I thought the idea was dead and buried and was fine with that, but I was mistaken, Kim had other plans.

We ended up purchasing a recumbent trike for me. Kim had thought of everything. It was a custom ride that was safe to operate even with bad balance. I was able to go out on solo adventures. The strange looks that I would get from the people I passed didn't deter me.

I had only had the tricycle a short while when I decided it was a lovely spring day, I should take it for a spin. I had only done three or four solo rides at this point, so it was a big deal to me to be out and about on my own.

We live in a hilly area of town, and I was still getting used to making gear changes. Somehow I managed to get the chain stuck, and the trike stopped in its tracks. I didn't know how to fix it, so I got off and pushed the trike up the steep hill back to a shopping area that I had passed. I knew there was a rack there that I could lock the bike up to until I could get ahold of Kim and have him fix it on his way home from work.

My plan was to strip the bike of anything that could get stolen and then wait for the next bus to come along. I hadn't realized that I had left home without any money. I was hovering between the bus stop and the bike when a young man approached. He looked to be in his twenties, tall and lean with stringy brown hair. He was dressed all in black, clothes that looked far too warm to be wearing for the weather that day.

I hoped that if I asked nicely he would be able to help me. I began to approach him when out of the blue he spat on me. What the hell! He didn't spit at me once; it was three times in rapid succession. I didn't think it was wise to provoke the situation, because I didn't know who or what I was dealing with. I was in shock. Thank God a bus approached, I wanted to get as far away from him as I could. Even though I didn't have the fare I explained what happened and the driver let me on.

The culprit likely never gave me a moment's thought, but I have thought of him though on occasion. I wonder what his life is like now, if he is still trying to get reactions out of people with his behaviour. I'll never know.

There was no explaining his actions. It just seemed to me that the more my health declined, the more I attracted unusual people and had peculiar encounters.

Even the simple act of walking along the sidewalk holding hands with Kim provoked a response from a passerby when I was unable to go at a pace that satisfied the couple behind us. I was slowing them down. How dare I be a hindrance!

As they walked by the woman said in a loud voice so that I would be certain to hear her. "Some people walk so fucking slow."

The man looked like he could take on anybody and easily win, so you think I would have kept quiet. I don't know what the hell came over me, instead of letting things go I answered back. I was acting completely out of character. Before I could really give it any thought, I replied, "You would walk slowly too if you had had a broken knee cap." It was the first thing that came into my mind even though it wasn't my knee acting up that day, it had been my neurological pain. They didn't need to know that.

Not wanting to give me the last word the woman said, "My legs are perfect, thank you," in a decidedly condescending tone.

I ended the matter by saying, "Then you are very, very fortunate." I am sure that Kim expected fisticuffs right there on the sidewalk, but I wasn't letting things go.

It stunned me when the gentleman had the decency to apologize to me on the lady's behalf. He grabbed the young woman, gave her the dirtiest look I had ever seen, and they quickly retreated into the closest store. I very much doubt that that was their intended destination. The fact is, situations like these happen every day throughout the world. Many of these encounters escalate into something serious, in a blink of an eye. Knives come out and guns get shot, and yet for that brief moment in time I didn't care. I was oblivious to the danger. I am thankful that the man took control and got the couple out of the situation.

The reason I had such an out of character response isn't entirely clear to me. I wasn't taking my customary sensible approach that I had come to rely on, I was standing my ground. I was even pleased with myself for doing so. Upon reflection I think this was the earliest warning sign that things were about to change. I had finally reached the point where I was going to rise up, get my pilot light stoked, and set the world ablaze. It was about time.

Part Two

stoking the flames

Let the Battle Commence

One blazing hot summer day turned out to be the pivotal moment when everything changed. We had been in the car for most of the day driving to visit family. We were on vacation a few hours away from where they lived and thought we didn't want to be that close without seeing them, so we took a day trip to meet them for lunch.

After having a wonderful day together, during our ride back to the hotel I noticed how incredibly swollen both of my legs had become. By the time we arrived back at our hotel room, they resembled tree trunks. They were so incredibly heavy and felt rock hard to the touch. It was as though my legs were going to explode because there was no more room under my skin.

This was a first for me, I had many medical ailments but swelling had never been one of them. I was lying on the bed questioning what the trigger might have been. Was it sitting in the car for too long, or the intense heat perhaps? I had plenty of questions running around in my head but no satisfactory answers. "How can my blood still be pumping? There didn't look to be any room left for the veins." I started to become anxious. What if the blood couldn't circulate? That could be deadly. I don't know the first thing about medicine. If I did, I certainly wouldn't have got myself into this predicament that's for sure. When I am anxious my mind goes to some pretty crazy places. Would I lose my legs? That might seem alarmist but lack of circulation doesn't allow for many options.

Because I have a somewhat warped sense of humour, I thought "Maria, you just can't lose any height. You are already short, you need to fix this, and urgently too." I was trying to laugh my way out of a tough situation, but all kidding aside, I knew it was time to get serious. The confrontation with the woman about walking too slowly was still fresh in my mind. The universe was obviously sending warning shots in my direction. Okay, universe you have my attention. I haven't got a clue what I should be doing, so if you insist on sending warning shots you better be sending me solutions while you are at it.

It was at that moment that I drew a line in the sand. I sternly said to myself that I could call it quits right now and wait for death, or buy some armour and find someone that could teach me how to battle. Those were my choices.

It was about two o'clock in the morning and I laid there in the quiet, listening to Kim sleeping peacefully beside me. I asked myself some pretty serious questions that night, things that needed to be asked.

What contributions had I made to get myself in this fine mess? What was I going to do about it?

What was I going to choose as my starting point to reclaim my life once and for all?

I made the decision that I was going to stop looking back,

stop living in the shattered mess my life had become, and focus only on reconstructing my life the way that I wanted it to be, one piece at a time.

After some deep thinking, I figured that I would settle at this point for not getting any worse. I couldn't rewrite history, but if I could stop the madness of my rapidly declining health, I would consider that to be a victory.

Okay then, I started to think, how can I stop myself from getting worse? The medical experts had ruled out just about everything. If a neurological professor didn't have the answer, what hope did I have? I had my work cut out for me.

It didn't come to me instantly, but sometime later that night, this voice inside me suddenly said, "Go to the gym." That was crazy. I must be imagining what I heard. Exercise had certainly never been my friend so why would exercising now be any different?

I suddenly had a flashback of an encounter I had had with a young man the last time that I had gone to the local recreation centre. I went for water walking because I thought that that might make me less wobbly. I was really unsteady on my feet and it was frightening me to death.

This particular day after water walking, I decided to go into one of the two other pools, in an open area that anyone could use. I wasn't in a specific swim lane so I wouldn't be interfering with anyone, besides, I had the area to myself. I am not a good swimmer. I can kick and kick and go nowhere. I was trying though, out there in the shallow end alone, bothering no one.

After only a few minutes, a young man whom I assumed was a lifeguard approached me. He said that I would have to get out because I wasn't swimming fast enough and the pool was for the swimmers. I was shocked into speechlessness. I wasn't interfering with anyone as there was no one close by. I wasn't in a designated swim lane, and if it was a public pool, wasn't I the public? What's his problem? If you want my opinion, the kid didn't want to have to keep an eye on me. He didn't want to do his job, and more than likely, he was enjoying what little bit of power he had been given. I was so accustomed to being treated badly by strangers that I just got out of the pool, got changed, and left without saying anything, even though I had paid to be there. What I should have done was tell the manager about this unacceptable behaviour. I wasn't particularly good at standing up for myself back then so it was just easier to remain silent.

What was I thinking! How could someone that can barely move go to a gym? It was a ludicrous idea. It was late, nothing was going to change overnight. I just needed to shut my eyes and get some sleep. I figured I would come to my senses in the morning.

The morning came and I still had that annoying voice playing in my head. "Go to the gym, you need to go to the gym." The thought just wasn't going away. Was this the universe's solution that I demanded they send me? I wasn't convinced of that yet. In fact, I spoke sternly to this inner voice: "Okay smartass, what gym? You know all too well that we have done that." The internal tug-of-war continued. I was either hallucinating or the voice said, "Then find one that works."

Because this thought wasn't going away, I actually decided to see if I could come up with some feasible solutions.

- Community recreation centres were out. Too crowded, lifeguards don't like me. Next...

- Go for a walk every day. Yeah, like that was going to happen. It hurts to move and I will probably fall. What do you mean by every day, exactly? Even the days that hurt? I must be mad. Next...

- Take up Tai Chi. You have to have balance for that, and my balance doesn't exist. Next...

- Use the stationary bike at home. Yep, but getting to it means going down the stairs that are really dangerous. The pitch is deadly, you have already fallen down them once, and have pins holding your ankle together to prove it. Do you want to go through that again just so you can use a boring bicycle? Next...

- What if you tried a regular gym rather than the rec centre this time? Yes, but they are filled with athletes. It's not meant for unfit people like me. Wouldn't I just be in the way? Next...

Man, my brain was relentless. I knew one way or another the voices were not going to subside until I was physically at a gym. I just hadn't resigned myself to that reality yet.

The road trip was strengthening my resolve to take action.

It was making me believe that there had to be an escape route. It was my job to find it. I hadn't considered an exit plan in over a decade. I might not be coming up with an idea that would work yet, but I had a drive in me that I had buried for a very long time.

This moment was my battle cry. My pilot light had dwindled to barely being an ember. I was existing, finding happiness wherever I could, but that is not the same as living. I hadn't lived in years. My ridiculously optimistic view of life was struggling to retain the smallest of flames. My body was done with living on hopes and dreams waiting to be rescued. No one was coming, it was the gym teacher leaving me alone on the trail all over again. There was no search party, I was it. I was my only hope, no one else, so what was I going to do about it? Failure was not an option. Start building that fire, we have work to do. Yes, I could feel the return of my inner spark start.

For some reason, I kept circling back to the concept of a gym. It just didn't seem like something I could see myself getting off of the couch for.

Although it wasn't quite right, I figured that if I fine-tuned it a little, it might be possible. I might actually be onto something.

Okay Maria, I thought, *if you don't want a commercial gym, what if you tried a hotel that has a gym for their guests to use? It would only be the fancier hotels that would include a gym, so there aren't that many for you to check. You could start there, you never know, they might even have a pool. One of them would probably let the public in, as long as you are willing to pay.*

That was one of the few times that I found myself doing some research on the internet. By the end of the day, I had settled on a nice local hotel with what looked like a fancy pool and more equipment than I could ever possibly know how to use properly. I let Kim in on what I was thinking and, bless his heart, he didn't laugh. I knew it would cost money and he was the one bringing in most of our funds. I told him that I just thought I wanted to try it. If it didn't work, and I honestly had given it a go, then I would just have to write the idea off. It was the only thing at this point though, that I could think of trying next.

The day after we got home from our family visit, we both went to take a look at the gym I had chosen. The hotel was lovely. The gym was in the basement, and I loved that I could hear myself think when we walked in. It didn't have eardrum-bursting music playing. There was music, but it was in the background where I thought it belonged.

I was excited that there was no smell of sweat. It was clean, bright and friendly. I was shocked that it didn't make me want to run for the hills. For a person that had avoided gyms and fitness for her entire life, that's a great start. There wasn't even the word 'gym' in their title. I could mentally trick myself into believing that I was just going to spend time hanging out at a fancy hotel. That should help get me there if I get desperate and willpower alone just isn't getting the job done.

Compared to the recreation centre, this place felt swanky. There was no need to bring change for the locker, as they provided lockers and towels to everyone as they came in. The fact that I didn't need to carry towels back and forth or need to wash them when I got home would make me feel like royalty. From the shampoo and conditioner, right down to complimentary apples: they literally had thought of everything. I didn't think I was going to find anywhere nicer. It was a perfect size, not too big that I would feel out of place, and yet it had everything.

The pool was a decent size for me, a non-swimmer, who couldn't drown in the deep end because my feet could touch the bottom. There was a whirlpool, sauna, steam room, you name it, it had everything. I would never in a million years use it all.

There were plenty of stationary bikes, treadmills, and the usual fare found at any well-equipped gym. There were even some ominous machines that definitely looked like they were meant for some sort of torturous pursuit. I didn't have a clue what any of these machines were for, mind you, and I wasn't intending to find out.

The people there were a wide spectrum of ages and abilities, each of them vibrant in their own way. From hotel guests with small children using the pool, corporate business types, and dedicated athletes, to those more advanced in years who just wanted to keep themselves moving. I could see myself fitting into that mix.

Down the road I could even look at taking one of their classes. There were tons of classes to choose from. What the heck is Pilates? Isn't Nia just a nice name for a girl, why is it up on the board as a class?

Someone around here obviously doesn't know how to spell either, because H I I T is spelled with one I, has no spaces or capitals, everyone knows that. I had so much to learn.

I had looked at the gym on the internet first and it lived up to the pictures I had seen on their website. I had already decided that if the place was nice, it would make committing to going regularly that much easier. It wasn't as though I picked several to show Kim. My inner voices were applauding me loudly.

I had only one concern, and that was that Kim might be thinking that, seeing as we didn't know if I would be able to physically stick to going to the gym, he could be leaning more towards trying the much less expensive option of the municipal recreation centre first. Then if I managed to keep going, we could think of upgrading to something like the hotel gym later. Fortunately for me, he thought I had gone through so much and deserved a nice place to come to.

The gentleman at the desk gave us a complimentary pass each and I returned the next day. Kim was at work, but I figured that was OK. I've got this. I'm the one who will need to come all the time. This was about me, no one else. I couldn't send a friend to exercise on my behalf. If the unbalanced, non-athletic, younger version of me could see me now, she would want to know what the hell I thought I was doing.

I was going to my edge and jumping. I was either going to crash land or I was damn well going to learn how to fly.

Ready or Not World, Here I Come

When I got home, I booked a ride with our local HandyDart service to go back to the hotel a few days later. The HandyDart service provides transportation for people who have difficulty using public transport. A small mini-bus picks you up at your home, takes you to where you want to go, and then comes back later to take you home. Being unsteady on my feet, I was eternally grateful that the drivers always made certain that I got safely to the place I was going including walking me to the door.

I had dug out some shorts, an old T-shirt to wear and I actually had to hunt for the running shoes that lived at the very back of the closet. I certainly didn't feel like I looked good in what I was wearing, but I knew gyms were never fancy dress. Once again, I reminded myself that people wouldn't notice, because they would just think that I was a hotel guest.

This time there was a lovely young lady at the desk who was very welcoming. The look of "what are you doing here?" that I had expected to see didn't happen. Instead, she smiled, assigned me a locker number, gave me a towel, and said that she hoped I had a good session.

I made my way to the change room and located my locker.

As I put away my purse, I was commending myself for being brave on one hand and telling myself that I didn't belong there on the other. Physically I was there, now I just needed to convince my mind to come along. These were the same inner voices that had only days before been persuading me to try the gym in the first place, so I decided to ignore any negativity. I took a deep breath, grabbed my water bottle, shut the locker behind me, and made my way out to the gym.

I stood there for a moment taking it all in, watching other people doing what looked to me like very athletic moves. I only briefly glanced as I did not want to appear to be staring at anyone. As I didn't know what most of the fancy equipment was for, or how to use them, I decided to stick with something I had at least used before—the exercise bike. There were a couple of different styles to choose from, but I figured I was safest with a recumbent bike to begin with.

I was fairly quiet that day. I sat on the bicycle trying to comprehend how to turn the machine on. After a few minutes, I adjusted the settings and settled in for a spin. As I sat there, I thought about my time with Pam and my neurological physiotherapy adventure. She would have been pleased to see me trying the gym but would have been saddened to discover that all the success we had achieved together had slipped away. I watched my feet slowly go around on the pedals. I was giving it my best effort, but the most I could manage was about 30 revolutions a minute. It was better than nothing, but it reminded me how difficult it was going to be to get my health back.

I had scheduled my outing to the gym for after my midday

prescription fix, thereby hopefully avoiding more pain, but it was usually that time in my day when I would be medicated to the point that I could nod off without warning. There wouldn't be a perfect time to go to the gym. I was either recovering from having taken my medication or gearing up for the next lot. I needed to decide that I was going no matter how I felt.

I noticed that some people were wearing headphones and thought that might be good for me, too. If I was just sitting there, not only would it help pass the time, but I could play a tune that would help keep me moving. I made a mental note to dig out my old iPod and headphones for the next visit.

A few people said hello or acknowledged my existence as they went past, which was nice. For the most part though, people were busy doing their own thing. I spent most of my time that day thinking about my decision to come to the gym, and if I was an idiot or a genius for doing so. I couldn't make my mind up. It was too early in the process to know.

As I got off the bike, I saw a row of treadmills and made a mental note to try them one day, once I thought I could safely get on and off the machines.

I had booked the HandyDart service to come back in an hour. I thought that would be more than enough for the first day. Because I was so out of shape, I only lasted about half an hour, but for me, that was a great first effort. I decided to call it a day and wait for my ride in the lobby.

That very day, I decided that if I was going to do this right, I wasn't going to do the drop-in thing. It would be too easy to make excuses not to come. I was giving myself as few escape clauses as I could, as my inner self really took matters into her own hands. I went crazy and got a one-year membership after only trying the place out for half an hour.

I figured that it was bound to take me at least a year to get better. I had committed to giving my idea a try, and I didn't even know if it would work. I had jumped over the cliff. Somehow that gym was going to become part of my everyday world if it killed me, and it just might.

That night when I got home, I told Kim all about my adventure. I was really proud of myself for going, but I reminded myself that this was only day one. If I meant what I said about getting better I was going to have to do it all over again tomorrow. I was physically exhausted; it had taken everything out of me to not only get there and back, but to work out as well. That was a heck of a lot of activity for one day. If you included getting ready, I did more activity that day than I would have done in an entire week normally.

I was in pain and felt completely knackered. I quickly fell asleep on the couch, and Kim woke me at nine o'clock because he knew it was time to take my medication. In my half-awake state, I crawled off to bed to call it a night. I was back asleep in record time and was sound asleep until Kim gave me my morning meds at five o'clock. There is something wrong when you are woken out of deep sleep to get medication that makes you sleepy.

If at First You Don't Succeed

I went to the gym every single day for an entire month, and sat spinning away on the bicycle. I didn't feel that I was spinning any faster, but over that month, I began to be able to ride for longer. The gym itself has several different areas to work out in, depending on what exercise you were doing. There was a big main section with most of the equipment in a row down the middle and along the edges. The weight area was tucked in one corner, then around the rest of the space was all the other big pieces of equipment. As I didn't know what the equipment was for, I ignored those machines completely.

You have to go through the big main room, pass the squash court and fitness studio, then around the corner to find the cardio room with the bicycles. It was a rather long and narrow space when you compare it to the rest of the gym. It was filled with a few treadmills, the upright and recumbent bikes, a couple of elliptical machines, some stair climbers, and a rowing machine. These were all there to get my heart pumping once I have built my stamina up to give them a try.

It had very large television screens attached to the wall on two of the corners. I figured they were there to help pass the time as you strolled on the treadmill or spun on the bike. I understand why the big TVs are popular, but in my opinion, they were a bit of overkill. If you want to watch anything, it had to be on mute, so you were either reading the closed captions or just watching the picture, so for me it felt like too much work.

One wall of the cardio room is primarily glass, providing a view of the swimming pool area. As I got more familiar with my fellow gym members, I would often see one of them wave at me or give me a thumbs up from the pool for moral support. That was really lovely. These had to be some of the nicest people that I have ever met. We share a common goal of being the healthiest we could be. I was mistaken to believe that gyms were the territory reserved for only the already physically fit among us. Here I was one of the unhealthiest people there and yet I was treated no differently than anyone else. I was starting to be recognized, and people often remembered my name. I felt safe in the cardio room because it was tucked away from everything else that was going on. I was protected on the bicycle because I could sit, strap my feet in and simply spin at whatever pace I managed to do that day.

I did begin to use the treadmill, but it was a far riskier proposition for me than the bicycle. Getting up on the machine wasn't impossible, but it was awkward. I would hang on to the side and hoist myself up. I placed myself perfectly between the two arms for support, making certain to connect myself to the safety line, that way I was assured the machine would stop if I started to wobble. In the very early days, the safety line saved me on quite a few occasions. With the machine set at barely moving and without any incline, I would begin.

Because I was unstable, even on solid ground, I found the treadmill to be a bit unsettling. I would only try it on the bravest of days. The fact that there was constant movement was more than enough to begin with. Getting off the treadmill was even harder than getting on was. I would slowly inch my way down while holding onto the side with all of my might. There was no graceful way for me to use a treadmill. I only kept trying because I figured that I needed to move.

On most days, I tried to put in an hour in the gym, give or take, but it took time to build up my endurance. I found that taking along music passed the time as I was spinning on the bicycle. It's boring just sitting there staring off into space, although I did get to see familiar faces and we would chat briefly. I would instinctively slow the pace of what I was doing in order to chat, so I welcomed each and every conversation. I was doing everything in my power to make this a success.

With considerable effort, I reached a whopping 40 RPM!!! On the bike, that was a big deal, even though it was at level one, and I couldn't sustain the effort for long, I was giving it a damn good try.

At the end of the month, I hurt as much as ever and the scale had yet to budge an ounce. It was a disappointment, to say the least. My efforts weren't being rewarded and I figured that a reward was definitely warranted. Clearly doing things on my own was getting me absolutely nowhere. It dawned on me: I'm going to have to go to a personal trainer for answers, aren't I? Oh, this is not going to be pretty. In football terms, this would be my hail Mary pass.

When you are in the depths that I found myself in, it would be the equivalent of going to Mount Everest with no prior climbing experience and expecting to successfully summit the peak on my first attempt without help. Like any good mountaineer knows, you can't do everything alone. They hire Sherpas as guides to getting them safely to the summit and back. It was time to go looking for my own Sherpa.

Included in my yearly membership was a complimentary hour with the trainer of my choice. Back to the internet I went to read about each of the potential trainers. It didn't matter to me one way or another if it was a man or a woman, as long as they could keep me from getting worse. As I was reading about each of them, I came across someone who I thought might work: Harley Preston. His biography said that he was a medical exercise specialist, among other things. I didn't know what a medical exercise specialist was exactly, but it piqued my interest. I theorized that because I had successfully stumped the medical profession, I had best go for a trainer with at least the word medical somewhere in their biography. Let's see if I stump him as well. I had yet to meet anyone that I didn't easily confuse when it came to my many medical ailments.

Everyone else's biography had a picture of the person with it, except for his. You can tell a lot about someone's personality from a picture. Seeing as his picture was missing, my guess was that either he didn't play by the rules or he wanted to be mysterious. I didn't know what I would be getting myself into. I took a deep breath and decided that, sight unseen, I would give Harley a try. I asked the front desk to set up my free session on my way out. What did I have to lose?

Unbeknownst to me, Harley happened to be just at the start of his vacation. I waited two weeks and heard nothing. I just thought he either wasn't interested or had lost my contact details. When I followed up on the matter, the receptionist suggested trying someone else. I did give it a brief thought only to decide that I would bide my time and wait for Harley. Some inner voice told me not to be an idiot. I had waited many years to take decisive action; another few weeks were not going to kill me.

Upon Harley's return, he called me to set up a time to meet. It was a holiday long weekend, and he said he could meet me on Monday. I was surprised that he would come in on a statutory holiday, but he said it didn't matter to him as he was well-rested from his vacation. That explained where he had been. I wasn't being ignored after all, which made me feel better. We agreed to meet early that Monday morning.

I was a mix of apprehension and excitement on the day. Not the "Oh boy!" kind of excitement, but the "Good for you" kind of excitement. I was taking action, taking control and it was about time, too.

When I arrived, I waited in the reception area. I had no idea who I was looking for, I only had the mystery man's name, Harley Preston. At the agreed-upon time, a young man approached me with a clipboard in hand: "Hi, I'm Harley."

He was pretty much what I expected, a very fit and confident young man somewhere in his mid-to-late thirties but I am not particularly good at guessing anyone's age. Honest to God, it was his smile that I noticed first, warm, friendly, and a wee bit mischievous. That being said, I would have had to be blind not to have noticed how incredibly fit he was. He was a slender man about five-foot-nine or so, with really deep brown eyes and thick dark hair that was perfectly in place. He looked strong and athletic. He was a perfect example of how a person would look if they worked out regularly and was his own best advertisement.

He didn't look like a stereotypical bodybuilding freak, though, with excessive bulging muscles, but I could tell that he knew his way around a gym. That's what I needed. Now that I could put a face to the name, I realized that I had seen him around the gym before, talking to various people, and had said hi a few times when I went by.

After completing some mandatory paperwork, he led me to a small, relatively quiet area of the gym where there was a comfortable padded bench for us to sit and get acquainted. In a quiet business-like tone he said, "Tell me about any health concerns I should know about."

Where do I begin? I thought to myself. I tried to get all of the important details in, but there was just so much to tell him. I could feel myself rushing, and in hindsight, it might have been easier just to tell him what was working well instead. It would have been a much shorter list. He really was opening the floodgates with that question. I bet he has never had anyone with such a complicated list as mine. Not that I was in any way proud of that fact, far from it.

Telling him what was wrong with me was akin to going to confession. I had to be completely, brutally honest with myself and with him if I stood any chance of getting my health back. I wanted that more than I had ever wanted anything else in my entire life. This hour was crucial, so I needed to make the most of every minute that I had with him.

At one point he was scribbling things down so fast that he was having trouble keeping up. I had to take a breath and slow down in order to give him an opportunity to get all the pertinent details down on paper.

I rattled off my medications like it was just another fact, because to me that was all it was, just another fact.

"That's some pretty heavy-duty medication you are on there," he said.

"Yes," I agreed, "and I am still in debilitating pain."

His response surprised me. "It would be nice to see you off of the medication."

That very second, a mental bolt of lightning struck me. I had never in all the years of dealing with my declining health, had anyone even suggest reducing my medication, never mind getting off of it entirely. He didn't know it, but I was pretty much sold right then and there.

He had only said it would be nice, but that was all I needed to hear. Naturally, he hadn't made any promises and certainly didn't give any indication as to how that would even be possible, but I wasn't asking those types of questions. I simply liked that someone I didn't know would like to see me off of my medications. Was it just a sales pitch? I would have to wait and see.

Most of that hour was just me babbling on about my health, or lack of good health to be more precise. With about 20 minutes left, he put a mat down and showed me some very simple stuff. I figured just getting up and down to the mat was exercise. This was only the beginning, I wasn't ready for proper exercise yet. Once safely on the ground, we started with some good deep breaths. A full inhale and then as complete an exhale as I could muster. So far so good.

Next, he had me lay on my back and bring my legs up to 45 degrees. Then I simply moved them slowly from side to side.

"I want you to just connect to what your body is doing and feel all the different muscles that are working to move your legs from side to side," he instructed. I could feel them alright!

Then he had me put my legs straight out and simply attempt to lift my feet two centimetres off of the ground, and hold them there without dropping my legs.

"Challenging isn't it?" I heard him say. He was completely right, but all I managed was some sort of grunt in reply. That seemingly simple move was absolutely a huge challenge for me. It reinforced what I had known for some time: just how low I had sunk, and how far I would have to go to get out of this mess. Those last 20 minutes of the session flew by.

At the end of the hour, Harley said to me, "If you want to work together sometime just let me know." With that, he shook my hand, gave me half a hug, then turned around and walked away. I certainly wouldn't call it a hard sales pitch, that's for sure. I had geared myself up to hear a hard sell. I wasn't quite sure what to do when that didn't happen.

There I was, he had all kinds of information about me, more than I had probably told anyone else other than Kim, and I knew nothing about him other than now having a face to the name and his contact details. He hadn't even told me what he thought he could do for me. Now what?

It was back to those inner voices again. "What do you do now kid? Think about this very carefully. You need someone, and that someone is probably him."

Was I just going to give up now, when I was barely even at the starting line of my sparkling new self-care plan?

Where were my questions? I had spoken for almost that entire hour, and hadn't asked any of the questions that I clearly should have, like how long have you been a personal trainer? What's your teaching style? What kind of professional success have you had with clients, and what experience did he have working with people in a similar condition to me? Not to forget the most important question of all, how would he contribute to my success? The questions were coming much too late.

What I hadn't told a living soul was that I honestly believed that I would only have the strength and determination to try rescuing my health once. If this didn't work, I knew I would believe what the specialists had said—nothing more could be done. It would be game over. The only thing between success and failure was the belief I had in myself. It was my pilot light telling me to give it one more try. One more try was all I was going to be able to muster.

It was critical to be taking positive action, yet, here I was stumbling at the starting gate as I watched Harley walk away. He was a complete stranger, I couldn't say, "Hi, I'm Maria. I am in atrocious health and you have one shot to get this right with me, or I will end up returning to the couch and wait for death." He would likely have run away and who could have blamed him.

I didn't tell him that I had everything riding on making this choice. He was unaware that I would work harder than anyone, as long as he showed me how to get well. It would be too much to put all that onto Harley's shoulders having only just met him. I would have to keep the urgency of my situation to myself for the time being.

It seemed like most recent visits to the doctor resulted in some warning or another about being at risk of more medical complications later if I kept going along the way that I had been.

The way that I saw it, sooner or later I would be hearing that the prognosis was bad and all they could do for me was give me more and more drugs. I couldn't let that happen. I might be at-risk, I'll give them that, but the warnings that they gave me never came with the necessary solutions.

There really weren't any other options unless I wanted to

interview other personal trainers. Obviously, my interviewing technique would need serious improvement if I was going to keep looking. Did I need to keep searching for a trainer simply because he didn't try to sell me on hiring him for the job? He had been very pleasant and professional, his own fitness level clearly demonstrated to me that he knew a whole lot more about the subject than I would likely ever know. There was also that one sentence he said about it being nice to be off medication that was still playing in my head, and I really, really wanted that.

Oh and don't forget he is a medical exercise specialist, I told myself. *Where would I find another one? Look, can you judge a man on a twenty-minute session on a mat? Of course not, Maria. Just quit waiffing, either stay on your own or grab onto this lifeline and hold on. Okay then, Mr. Fit it is, it's decided.*

I felt relieved to have made a decision. It was a huge weight off of my shoulders. Maybe now those inner voices would stop pestering me.

I was smart enough to realize that I hadn't gotten in my current state overnight. Some of my conditions were from birth, while others had compounded over time. It was only fair to allow a few months before expecting any changes. I was going to put my future into Harley's hands. I paid for more sessions with him on my way out. I e-mailed him to thank him when I got home and arranged for our next session. I didn't know that I had just made a decision that would make my current life unrecognizable.

Gym Life

Fortunately for me, Harley isn't a man who backs down from a challenge. He loves stuff that makes him think. Anyone looking at me would know that I was far from fit, so this wasn't news. I could possibly be his biggest professional challenge to date. He didn't seem phased by that though, thank God!

He didn't know if I was going to be someone that really committed to getting better, or just another client who gives up when the work gets too tough. I would need to show him that I was worth investing his time and talents into. I didn't see a ruler for him to hit me with, and his pen looked pretty harmless, so Harley appeared safe. I was as ready as I would ever be, the question remained, was he?

Welcome to the world of gym life. The early sessions with Harley were primarily doing exercises on the mat, similar to those I had done that first day, each carefully crafted to exercise a specific muscle or muscle group. He always included a spin on the bike. The way he made me work on the bike was quite a bit different from what I had been doing on my own. I had always just continued to spin at whatever rate I could, and then if I needed a break or some water to drink, I would stop, take a sip and then start peddling again.

Harley had a different plan. He wanted me to spin as fast

as I could comfortably and then take breaks, but instead of stopping, I had to keep spinning the wheels while I allowed my body to recover. He frequently asked me how I was feeling and then had me do a heart rate check.

There were some pretty high numbers in those early days. I was working flat out, and yet the movement should be simple. Yes, he wanted my heart rate up, but not to dangerous, heart attack- or stroke-inducing levels. He is fully trained in first aid, but I didn't want him to have to spring into action on my behalf. I wondered why he didn't take my word for it when I said I was fine, but what I came to discover was that, how we think we feel, and how our body is actually feeling, sometimes differs.

For some peculiar reason, I often didn't register a heartbeat when I did a heart rate check with the sensors on the workout equipment. Obviously, I am breathing, but as far as the machine goes, I don't have a pulse. I would turn to Harley and say something smart like, "See, I'm heartless," or "Look, Harley, you have managed to break my heart." We would have a good chuckle even though I am sure he has heard it all before. There was no stopping, other than when I needed to physically recover or grab some water to drink. Harley was on a mission and he didn't skip a beat.

By the end of each of our sessions, even though I hadn't done much really in the scheme of things, I was exhausted. I continued to make myself go to the gym five times a week, taking two days off to be with Kim on the weekend, and let my body recover. I looked at going to the gym as my job. I was too unhealthy to work outside the home, so my singular focus was to get myself better.

I had only seen Harley a handful of times when he suggested that in addition to our private sessions I should come along to his gentle fit class. I saw on the event board that he offered several different classes throughout the week but never considered myself capable of going, or more importantly, surviving it. It wasn't a sales pitch, as classes were free with membership.

I wouldn't have normally gone along because things like that remind me of gym class, and those classes were something that I have always tried to block out of my mind. I didn't need flashbacks. In this case, though, Harley was well aware of my many limitations and would be less likely to try and make me do something I couldn't do. Staying firm to my commitment to embrace this whole process, I went along with his recommendation.

I made a point of arriving early, in hopes that I could position myself to be by the wall so that I could hold on if I needed to. The gentle fit class is something of a misnomer. It might get you fit but it wasn't particularly gentle. At least it didn't appear that way to me when I was at the beginning of my recovery.

That may relate to how extremely unfit I was. The class itself was held in the large studio space, and there was enough room for about twelve people to spread out with their mats and follow along. That first time, there were about eight of us all of them mature women of various ages, each one friendly and welcoming. Some of them might be older, some younger, but one thing was certain, I was the most inexperienced based on my history and the fact that I had not been in a gym class since high school.

This time I was there willingly, and I certainly wouldn't be ignored. There was a choice of a thin yoga mat or thick cushiony workout ones for people to use. I immediately gravitated to the thick ones as they would provide a higher degree of comfort and were probably much better for my bad knee. I could get up and down, but it was challenging. I would put both of my hands down for support, then bend my bad leg, and lower myself carefully. I just hoped that I didn't have to do it too often.

Class was a great continuation of what Harley and I had been doing privately. He had much more opportunity to work on breath technique and try a few things I hadn't done before. The first half-hour was easy because I was learning all about relaxation techniques. Who doesn't want to be good at being able to relax? It's a good job that my medication hadn't quite fully kicked in yet by the time class started as his quiet, calming voice would have put me to sleep in an instant. Instead, my neurological zaps were keeping time with the meditative music he had playing quietly in the background.

The second half of the class was action stations. I was a little out of my depth to be honest because I hadn't been able to do the exercises he was demonstrating. That didn't hold Harley back from including me in the class, though. As it happened, I was the only new kid on the block that particular day. He got the regulars doing something that they were accustomed to, and then he would alter the exercise to my level, show me quickly how the simpler version needed to be done, and then watch over me to make certain that I was doing it properly. Once he was satisfied with what I was doing, he returned his attention back to the rest of the class and continued on.

He quietly assured me that day that I would eventually get it if I just kept coming to his class. His words of encouragement meant a lot to me. One of the things I found out later that he says often is, "Don't worry about getting it. Get rid of any outcome fixations and just be in the moment." I wasn't getting any of it, but as he said, I wasn't supposed to worry about that. It sounded like a foreign language to me, but it was enough to get me to come back the next week and most weeks ever since.

My fellow classmates cheered me on. This was a far cry from the gym classes of my youth. It didn't matter that we were all at different fitness levels. Harley took control and made us all feel capable of achieving whatever exercise he was requesting. He was serious about doing things properly but we all had opportunities to enjoy ourselves while we were doing it. Even if it was uniting in the opinion of what a taskmaster he could be. He took our comments in good stride which was exactly how we intended them to be. We were having fun with him and wouldn't be there if we didn't want to be.

I began by meeting with Harley once a week for an hour and then taking his gentle fit class once a week for an hour. The rest of the time I would go to the gym and work out on my own. The travel back and forth, along with the workouts, was all that I could do on a gym day. Once I got home, it was back to the couch until bedtime. It felt good to be out of the house for something other than a medical appointment. Fortunately, the class time worked well for my methadone doses once I settled into the routine. Even though it was all that I could manage, it was a worthwhile accomplishment. It was much better for me than sitting at home alone watching the television in my usual medicated state.

I did uncover an interesting fact that during time with Harley, although I could still feel the pain, it never got to the level that I would let out an involuntary scream. Thank God. Could you imagine if I had! That would have been so embarrassing. I might never have gone back. There was some grimacing going on, to be sure, but I don't think anyone was paying attention. If they did, they didn't say anything to me about it.

Each time I met with Harley, he did something that kind of freaked me out, just a little until I eventually became accustomed to it. He would look me in the eyes and ask me how I was, then actually wait for my response.

Who does that?! It sounds silly now that I put it down on paper, but that never happened to me. People ask how you are all the time almost without realizing it. It's all part of the word hello isn't it? It's not just "hello," it's "Hello, how are you?" Are people really asking me how I am? Usually not. I would like to think that it's just me, but I have had people walk away while I have been in the middle of responding to them. They either hadn't realized that they had even asked how I was, or weren't expecting me to say anything in response.

What Harley had done by waiting for me to answer him was force me to take a moment and think about how I was actually feeling and put it into words. It was the first reintroduction to my own body. I had to acknowledge how I was feeling in order to be able to answer him, a simple "fine" was not what the man was waiting to hear.

Harley is all about paying attention to your body and what it is telling you. When people would ask how I was I had become programmed to just automatically say, "fine thanks." It was an automatic response to an automatic question. I wasn't fine, far from it, yet the words just came out of my mouth without any thought required. Now I had to specifically think about how I was and verbalize it. It seems that I might be dealing with a freak of nature; Mr. Fit might just be a creature from another planet entirely.

Even just doing the beginner stuff, along with his class, soon began showing results. Within a couple of weeks, I was already strong enough to remove the bed rail that I had been relying on for a couple of years.

Hallelujah! That was pretty darn impressive. It was the first positive health result I had had since seeing Pam, and in such a relatively short amount of time too. I thought to myself, *Wouldn't it be wonderful if I saw results as I had with Pam, but this time keep going?* I tried not to get my hopes up, as it seemed too much to ask for, but I just couldn't help myself.

Harley had emailed me a list of exercises to start with, which I have named my Harley Knows Best List. Each time I was at the gym by myself I would religiously do the list in its entirely. I guess what I was doing looked like nothing at all to some of the fitter folks at the gym because one day I was working away at my list beside this younger woman who looked really sporty. She was finished before I was, and as she left, she turned to me and said, "Happy sleeping." I didn't respond, but I had an overwhelming urge to tell her that I wasn't sleeping. I was exercising, see!!! It's right here on my Harley Knows Best List.

Even though I wasn't specifically watching everyone else, there have been times when I have seen people do something amazing and I have stopped what I was doing to watch and simply admire their abilities. Sure, Harley can make any movement he has shown me look simple and effortless, but I think the most impressive thing I have ever seen while at the gym, was a young man do a handstand against the wall and then raise and lower himself. He had such control. When he was done, I felt compelled to tell him how impressive that was. I couldn't imagine even doing a headstand, never mind having the ability to be able to move up and down while balancing on your hands.

I learned early on not to pay attention to what anyone else was capable of doing. If I started doing that I would have said to myself, "What is the point, I'll never get there," and it would be game over. I turned a blind eye to what was going on around me and strictly worked on trying to do everything on my Harley Knows Best List as well as I could, and hopefully better than I had done them the day before. It was just that simple, nothing more than that. I paid attention to everything Harley was teaching me. What's the point of having a professional show you how to do something, then not at the very least try to do it the way you have just been taught?

Fun and Games

I kept a low profile in the early months, primarily because I didn't want well-intentioned people to ask me how things were going and watching my every move. There were only a handful of people who knew that I was on a mission. That way, no one would be any the wiser should I fail, even if that wasn't the plan.

There are pros and cons to this approach that I weighed very carefully. The more people who know, the bigger the cheerleading team I would have. That can be beneficial; however, I liked the simplicity of keeping my cheer crew very tight. They know who they are and that is all that matters. I didn't need to make it a spectacle, all I needed was success. I was my own secret agent. My plan was to tell people once I had anything great to report.

I was doing well enough after three or four months, that I could safely add an additional personal training session each week with Harley along with his strength and core class without any serious consequences. As a complete novice, the two classes seemed quite similar at first glance, but it was explained to me that the exercises we did during the stretch and core class worked different muscles than what we did during gentle fit. Taking both classes enabled me to have a more well-rounded level of movement.

Harley approached my introduction to his strength and core class exactly the same way that he had done with gentle fit. He would meet me where my ability was on that particular day, never pushing me past my limits. He would redesign the exercises as needed so that I had a safe starting point, and then slowly began coaxing me forward until I could do his more difficult version. It was pretty much the same group of people for both classes, with only a slight variation depending on people's schedules. They were accustomed to seeing me now and came to expect that I would be there in my usual spot. What a difference from my youth, this time I fit right in, and I looked forward to going.

Harley had warned me that customarily, people go along well at first when they are doing a new exercise program only to experience some sort of hiccup which he anticipated happening anywhere between a few weeks to a few months into the new routine. It's usually caused by overdoing things or perhaps pulling a muscle. This creates a new ache or pain to contend with. He loves to say that, "When muscles start to work correctly for the first time, you meet some unique inhabitants of your body along the way." You wake up dormant regions that prefer to remain undisturbed. Certain areas of the body insist on demonstrating their displeasure by acting up. It's nothing major, so I shouldn't be alarmed when it's my turn. According to him, it would probably only last a week or two if I am lucky before things got back on track. He assured me, however, that whatever happened I should be fine as long as I stuck to my Harley Knows Best List.

Thanks for the heads-up Harley, but as it turns out that didn't happen, much to my astonishment I defied the odds and somehow managed to escape any hiccups. Knowing how bad my health was, I had myself convinced that it was just a matter of time before "the inhabitants" revealed themselves. I kept what he had told me in the back of my mind in case something happened, but eventually it escaped my thoughts entirely.

I think it took quite a while for Harley to relax and stop expecting the e-mail or call to let him know I had injured myself—and much longer for me to let go of the sense that something bad might happen. Harley had put himself on high alert waiting to spring into action to get me through a setback. Sometimes when you are in an attack mode, you don't realize that the danger has passed and that you can settle down to the task at hand. He managed to keep me injury-free and added new exercises quite often to my Harley Knows Best List.

I saw Harley at the reception desk one day on the way out of the gym and was pleased as punch to report to him that, if I really pushed myself hard enough, I could get above 50 RPMs on the bike now and hold it for a moment or two. Then he confirmed my belief that he was from another planet.

"I don't want you to do that," he announced.

I was in a state of shock, and you could have blown me over with a feather. "What kind of personal trainer doesn't want me to go faster?" I asked.

He smiled and explained that it isn't all about pushing beyond your ability, it's about building your ability to do more difficult things easily. I gave him a big smile, shook my head in disbelief, and said, "Yes, dear," as I exited. What more was there to say?

Over time I realized that Harley didn't seem to be taking any exercises off of the list. Once the exercise was placed on my to-do list, it remained there. This meant that the amount of time I was spending at the gym to complete my routine kept getting longer. I was convinced that it was a sinister plot on his part to make things more challenging. He was succeeding on that score. He likely hoped that I somehow wouldn't notice what he was up to. I was aware of his shenanigans, I just didn't say anything because I knew that there was a probability that he would just add even more exercises if I brought the matter to his attention. I certainly didn't want that.

I came to realize that, although things were pretty much the same on the pain front, while I was focused on doing the exercises themselves, the pain did seem more manageable somehow. It could be that I was concentrating so hard on everything that I was doing that I managed to block out the pain. I don't have any idea what was causing this, but it was a great incentive to keep coming to the gym.

I could tell you each of the exercises Mr. Fit had me do, but this isn't an exercise manual, and I would be afraid that what works for me might not be the right combination of movements for someone else. The exercises themselves are always the same, but which ones to use, when, and for how long are a custom fit.

I learned that a lot of physical issues that we develop over time have to do with compensation patterns our body develops because different muscles take over, when the muscle that we should be using is either too weak or lazy to get the job done. I hear Harley say all the time that "work" is all about finding our weaknesses and turning them into strengths.

To do that isn't as simple as I would have hoped. You have to get the overworked muscles to stop what they are accustomed to doing, get the lazy ones to join in, and do their proper function. If things are functioning as they are meant to there are no free rides. When everything works harmoniously accomplishing whatever task you want to do should seem effortless.

I have never given myself a deadline for becoming fit. I find that whenever I have a deadline, all I think about is how much time I have, until I can get back to normal or how many more pounds need to come off so that I can stop dieting. I wasn't going to allow myself to feel fit and then think I was done. Gym life and working out needed to be a forever thing. If I let my eye off the prize, I could soon be back to visiting specialists—and that was something I dreaded.

In order for this monumental mission to work, I couldn't think about how much I hurt or how I could potentially reward myself for going to the gym once I got home. I had to be right there in the moment. Instead of complaining about going, I started to look at what a gift it was to be off of the couch. After all, I was that same woman who thought that it was a good day when I made it from the bed all the way to the kitchen. I would remind myself of that fact often.

Success can be as much a mental state of mind as it is about physical abilities. I find that if we decide something isn't going to work, we are absolutely correct. We might as well move on to something else right then and there. I had to believe this was going to work. I had no choice, I had run out of options. I didn't have a backup plan.

If I was going to have to work hard, I was going to make sure that Harley and I were both going to have some fun while we were doing it. Why would I keep seeing him and working out together if I dreaded it? That would make me quit, and then I'd be back on the couch believing that all that was left for me was death. That would never do.

There were times that I thought Harley had lost the plot and I would burst into fits of laughter. He would want me to contort my body to do a movement that was completely foreign to me.

What the heck was he thinking? He couldn't be serious. I wasn't trying to audition for Cirque du Soleil. I can't even do a tuck and roll. If I appeared reluctant, he would smile and then wait for me to do what he had requested. He wouldn't let me pick and choose what activities I did or didn't do. He was focused, I'll give him that. He wouldn't be deterred from whatever he had planned for me during our sessions unless there was a physical reason why.

It wasn't all his-way-or-the-highway, far from it. He soon

The Pilot Light Effect

got to know what moves I enjoyed or could do better than others, and would be sure to add them in, particularly if we were nearing the end of a session. It always felt good when we could end on a high note.

I always gave each exercise a try, and usually failed miserably at first. All I could do was laugh. I had to get over feeling embarrassed, mad or frustrated, and find a way to keep going.

I wasn't going to become an athletic sensation, so I was competing only against myself. In the scheme of things, I would often execute a move poorly and be thrilled to bits because it was the best I had ever done, or my first attempt at something, making me pretty impressed with myself.

Periodically someone would walk past us and say that we were having too much fun to be working out, but I think they were jealous.

The gym tends to be a serious place, all about how much weight you can lift or how many push-ups you can achieve. Then there was Harley and I giving each other a high five for "almost" doing something right, or me doing a happy twirl because even though it wasn't good it was better than the last time I tried. We were a contradiction to the norm, but then I have never claimed to be normal.

Harley continued to put the word "personal" in personal trainer, and I soon understood the value of that approach. I had only been able to survive his classes because he customized the exercises for me until I could catch up with the other participants. I loved the fact that he included everyone regardless of individual capabilities. It was an unusual sensation to be fully involved in a gym class rather than being on the sidelines, and I liked it.

Harley has got me so far out of my comfort zone that my workouts should have their own postal code. In my head, I would be convinced that I can't do this. *I am going to hurt myself... he's trying to kill you... I should run while I can.*

A few times I was physically shaking, knees knocking, and trembling uncontrollably, but I never turned down his requests to at least try the movement that he suggested, even if I thought about it more than once. I was afraid that if I said no, he would make me do something twice as hard as the exercise I was trying to avoid. He has more power than he lets on. Even though technically I am his client and the customer is always right, if I challenged him to a match of wills, I would come out the loser. I have never put that to the test as I don't want to be proven right.

One time in particular stands out to me as being beyond my comfort level. Harley was trying to get me to balance on top of an unsteady surface (Bosu) and squat with only a pair of cables to hold on to, the move wasn't going well. I was in an open space away from any walls for security. Even holding on to the cables Harley had set up for me didn't stop me from swaying wildly while trying to balance. I was smiling when I told him that if I fell he was going to be fired.

Harley isn't a fool, he doesn't want anyone to be injured. He was standing inches away, ready to catch me if I needed it. Even with him as my bodyguard, I was never so scared in my life as I was in that moment, not even when I got lost along the trail or was trapped in the bed beside Bernice. This was an entirely different type of fear. Those other times I was scared by the situation, but this fear came from me believing that my body was ill-equipped for the situation I was in.

I have always been aware of the fact that I am completely vulnerable when it comes to my balance. My lack of balance has been debilitating for my entire life. I don't have a built-in safety mechanism, everything is scarier. I spend a great deal of time and energy just trying to avoid dangerous scenarios. My life can be compared to continually walking through a minefield, watching every step you take, making sure you can get from one side of the field to the other without being blown up. I am in a permanent state of alert, and I have to be.

I have conquered many challenges, but my lack of balance is by far the toughest obstacle I am likely to ever have. There is a saying that you never miss what you have never had. That just isn't true. I have never experienced what it is like to have perfect balance, and yet I can clearly see how different my life is because I don't have it.

When Kim was six, he saw his older brother riding a two-wheel bicycle, he asked if he could try, got on, and immediately rode without anyone showing him how to do it. He wasn't even wobbling, there were no training wheels or hours of instruction beforehand—he had natural ability. I can only imagine how it would feel to be that fearless.

I have a long list of what I can and can't do when it comes to balance. This was most definitely at the top of things I shouldn't be doing.

That's why I believed that I was in great danger that day at the gym and simply panicked. Although I was attempting not to scream, an involuntary one came out. We stopped once that happened and we have never tried to do that move since. Perhaps he was wanting to test my limits. We had reached my limits and more with that move.

Harley did get scientific on occasion when he is going over the names of muscles he wanted me to fire for example, and I find it can go in one ear and out the other. Even though I am listening to him at the time, I just can't retain what he is saying, so I ask him to please translate that into "Maria." He has become quite fluent in "Maria," which is just as well because you can't find a Google translation between the scientific lens that he sees the world through and my need for keeping things simple. When you are learning things from the ground up there is an amazing amount of detail that you need to take in. Sometimes I find that it just becomes a bit overwhelming.

I don't always understand the reason we do things the way we do. I just do them because Harley tells me to and in the order he tells me to do something in. When he is trying to stress the importance of what he is showing me, his tone changes and everything becomes just that little bit more dramatic. It is his change in tone that makes me sit up and take notice.

What we do together can get intense at times, but if you can put a fun spin on things you still learn what you need to in order to remain safe and injury-free. Whenever you see people that are having fun, it's human nature to want to join in. I call it our fitness fiesta. As long as it gets me to the gym, there is a reason to party.

I am not what you call a cookie-cutter client. Because I had no concept of what I was doing, I didn't seem to fit the usual expectations. With a lot of exercises, I think it was almost beneficial not to have done them before. Harley didn't have to get me to stop doing something a certain way and correct it. He could show me how to do things properly right from the start.

What most people could do with relative ease I couldn't. I think Harley had to throw out his rule book and make a new one up. Rules are meant to be broken, and we were going to write our own from scratch.

I Can't Wait Forever for Your Approval

Once I noticed that I could help my pain levels while exercising, my inner voices became very vocal again.

Remember what Harley said that very first day? He's right you know, it would be so nice to see you off of the medication. You want that. Why don't you see if you can come off of them and find out if you can cope without them?

Much like before it became like a broken record playing over and over again in my head. It had such a taunting tone. It wasn't going to go away until I took some sort of positive action on the matter.

The next time that I saw Dr. Welsh, I told him about what happened with my pain levels while I was exercising and asked if we could cut my medication down because I wanted to see if I could cope with less medicine now that I was exercising. He wouldn't hear of it. He was absolutely right when he pointed out that we had spent years experimenting to get something that would even touch the pain that I was in. I had complex medical issues beyond just pain. It was a delicate balance keeping me going. I had been dependent on the drugs I was now so determined to eradicate for many years, was it any wonder then that he wasn't on board.

Although it wasn't the answer I wanted, I respected his judgment because he is a health-care professional. I reluctantly carried on taking the medication while continuing to do my exercises with Harley. The thought never completely left my head, though. The voices eventually went quiet, but I knew I hadn't heard the last of them.

I would not dream of taking matters into my own hands and just come off of prescription medication without discussing it first with my doctor. It was something too serious to mess around with, so I was trying to find a way to get Dr. Welsh on board with what I wanted to do.

If you are reading this and think it is a brilliant idea to just stop taking prescribed medications of any sort without medical supervision, you are wrong and could even be dead wrong. Do not do it under any circumstances. The only reason I am including this will soon become apparent.

Over the coming months, I asked Dr. Welsh a few more times if I could try and work towards coming off of my medications, always getting the same answer. He had not altered his original opinion that I needed to continue with things the way that they were.

I started imagining the steps I needed to take in order to reduce the medications, sometimes even allowing myself to imagine what it would feel like without them at all. It is out of character for me to go against medical advice, but in this case, I thought it was the only way to know how I was doing. I didn't think that the pain was going to stop, but if I could handle the pain without taking medication, surely that would be a better alternative.

Kim knew what I was thinking and cautiously went along with me on the matter. Whenever I figured it was time to approach the subject with Dr. Welch again, I would tell Harley, and he would patiently wait to get the latest update after my appointment. Harley had invested heavily in my success by this point and I thought he should be in on what I was planning next.

In a last-ditch effort one day, I assured Dr. Welsh that if coming off of my medications didn't work, I would take full responsibility for anything that happened. I would go back to my current doses without complaint and that would be the end of the matter. I wouldn't bug him about it again. Of course, I had no idea that when you are on the medications that I was taking, getting off of them was in fact a big deal. There was a real possibility that I could have a stroke or other serious medical complication. That would be a whole new medical nightmare, all for the sake of an experiment.

I had asked him several times by this point about lowering my medications, so I think he knew if he didn't tell me how to do it, I might go rogue on him and do it anyway. That day he said, "If a person were to come off of the medicines that you are on, it would have to be done this way..." It wasn't exactly a ringing endorsement, but I took it as a reluctant tutorial. I will leave it up to your own imagination about what I had planned if he had continued to resist my request. He was only trying to keep me safe, but I can be pretty determined when I set my mind on something. It's good that he gave me the tutorial because it wasn't at all the way that I had envisioned. The order that things needed to be done was completely different from what made sense to me.

What we never discussed was the withdrawal and what to expect. I figured it was going to be tough going, but even though I knew I had to be careful, I don't think that I was as prepared as I thought I was, or as aware of the danger as I needed to be. Dying was a possibility and yet it just seemed to be another word to me at the time. After all, wasn't I already dying inside a little bit more with each passing day? To be fair, I didn't ask Dr. Welsh to explain the effects of withdrawal to me, so it is in no way his fault that I didn't know. In hindsight, it was probably best that I was somewhat clueless. If I had researched the matter, I would have lacked the courage to go through with it.

Because my doctor was only at the reluctant tutorial stage, I never gave him the courtesy of saying that I was going to get off of the methadone come hell or high water. I therefore didn't have anyone supervising the actual withdrawal process. That would have been sensible! I figured that I was seeing the doctor every week anyway, and there was always the hospital emergency department if things got bad. It wasn't as though I was going off into the woods alone, to get the job done.

Instead of a medically supervised withdrawal, I'm out there on my own in the sense that I was the only one living through the physical reality of my situation, not knowing if what I experienced was normal, or something that I should be alarmed about. I might as well have been walking a tightrope suspended 150 feet in the air over a pit of ravenous crocodiles, and you know by now how good my balance is. As you see all the time on the television when something dangerous is about to happen: **do not try this at home.**

Sadly, I know a lot about pain and its power. Yet I don't know the first thing about the psychological and physical power of medication on the body when you try to part ways with it. Opiate withdrawal was light years away from what I was accustomed to. I was about to experience hell on earth: self-inflicted detox.

With the reluctant tutorial freshly playing in my mind, I knew that this was the time to go for it. I knew I couldn't wait for things to be perfect. Things might never be perfect. That night as I attempted to sleep, I felt the full weight of the chains that had been holding me back. Hold on just one more night, I told myself. Tomorrow my pilot light will begin to shine that little bit brighter until it can once again be the flame I have been searching for.

My cheerleading crew knew about going to the gym and working out with Harley, but the only people who knew about the upcoming withdrawal stage of the adventure were Kim and Harley. I trusted them both not to say anything to anyone and they both kept their word. It was a top-secret mission.

For everyone's safety, I can't tell you the specifics of what I did or how I did it exactly, other than to say I cut back my dose at set times and at set intervals until I was on a small enough dose to be able to stop completely. If you are reading this, and want to do something similar, please see a doctor so that he or she can advise you based on your individual circumstances.

What I can share with you is what it felt like. It wasn't just one bad night. I couldn't say to myself, "Suck it up princess, you'll be fine in the morning." Kim handed me a bucket and said, "You are going to need this." He was right: it didn't take long for the vomiting to begin and in this case, it was unavoidable. I hung on to that bucket like a lifeline.

My body was just beginning to express how angry it was to be going through such torment. While in the throes of withdrawal, it felt as though I was possessed by millions of insects crawling throughout my body. I could feel them scurrying through my veins. Meanwhile, others were burrowing into my heart and lungs. They were inside my eyelids, and slithering along every single hair follicle as well as wrapping themselves around each individual brain receptor. There was nowhere that didn't take a hit. My body was a war zone.

My marrow was being replaced by the creatures, or so it seemed. It felt as though my skin became paper-thin as it struggled to contain the invasion. This thin sheath was all that protected me from meeting my enemy face-to-face. If I got as much as a paper cut, I was convinced that the insects would begin oozing out, taking with them my last breath. My bones felt as though they had been gnawed away from the inside out. It was as though every bone could turn into dust at any moment. My chest was being squeezed ever tighter, leaving it to feel like a shriveled mass. Although it lessened in intensity over time, the insect invasion stayed with me for months.

My body began performing random involuntary twitches. Sweat was the only thing that managed a successful escape. I was restless, I would pace like a caged animal during the night. I was going back and forth between the sofa, the spare bedroom, and our bed. It didn't matter where I was, the insect invasion came with me. I would last perhaps twenty minutes at each place, throw the pillow on the ground, and head for the next spot, only to have the same result.

I was desperate for sleep or death—either would do. My body dismissed my requests. I had caused the mayhem within, and I wasn't going to be let off the hook for causing such devastation. I had a front-row seat to the fracas that was going on inside me. There was no escape.

This continued for months. Through it all, Kim stood watch. He felt pretty powerless because he couldn't physically make things better. Emotionally though, he made a colossal difference. He made endless cups of tea, made sure that the house was clean, and that I was fed. He took on so much to make sure that I had the best chance of success. My sole responsibility was to persevere and get through this ordeal safely. As the insects dominated, he would hold me tight and will me to keep going.

Harley checked in often and would send e-mails of support. He took great care of me whenever I was at the gym. Even if I hadn't booked time to work out with him, whenever he would see me at the gym, he would make a point of quietly asking how I was doing. I was so thankful that they were both there looking out for me. I didn't feel the least bit smothered. They just needed to give me the space to work through it all in my own way. They were simply willing to help should I need it.

I was in turmoil like never before. I didn't think my body was ever going to forgive me, and I couldn't blame it. Over time I became inwardly angry. I could feel the fire of hell. I kept replaying the fact that this had all started by seeing my doctor about unusual pains in my left leg. Years later, I am still in a crap avalanche of health troubles. Now here I was clawing my way out of the chasm, without a safety net, hanging on by my fingertips trying not to lose ground.

When a person takes a pill to relieve their back or headache, the toxin doesn't go just to those areas, it might make that particular area pain-free, but it travels throughout the body on the way down to the area in question. I had many years of polluting my body. I was paying the price. My body couldn't care less if the drug is illegal or prescribed. It was processing what I had been feeding it. When you take something for years, your body is like a two-year-old having a temper tantrum the moment the withdrawal takes hold.

The medication had made itself quite at home inside me, like a permanent house guest. My body had become quite accustomed to the company. They had developed a harmonious co-existence until I decided I needed to take control and break up the party.

Because the effects of my medications were throughout my body, it felt as though every inch of me had declared war simultaneously. I was a singular warrior princess against the enemy. It's almost impossible to be victorious when that enemy is yourself.

At the epicentre of the ordeal, I desperately wanted some sense of peace. I knew I still had some methadone in the fridge. Why in hell was I doing this? Really, what the holy hell was I thinking? The magic elixir was waiting just a few feet away in the fridge. I could imagine it trickling down my throat, as it negotiates the ceasefire that I had been longing for. Who do I think I am, coming off of such an addictive substance without the doctor right beside me every step of the way. No one even told me I had to come off medication in the first place. I certainly wasn't out to try and impress anyone. No one in the world would blame me for going back on the medication. It would be considered a valiant effort. That should be enough. For me, it would be settling for a silver medal, and I wanted gold.

Many people would have thrown away the medication so they wouldn't be tempted, I didn't. You see, the way I looked at it, if the medication was there, that would prevent me from feeling desperate. I would be the one in control. I needed to be at the helm of the command centre on this mission in order to ensure success. If I really couldn't do this, I could pull the plug at any point, and probably within a few days my body would have acclimatized and life would go back to how it had been. But that life was what I had been trying to escape so why would I settle for going backward? I couldn't do that, the only way to go was forward.

Once again my voices became vocal. *Maria, if you don't come off the medication you are going to be dead. Listen to me! Dead is forever. What if this is your only shot? This one right here, this very night. If you give in now, you will end up taking even more medication, you will still be in pain, and you will welcome death when it comes as a reasonable alternative. That isn't you.*

Believe in yourself, even though you don't understand why you are going through all of this. Remember what Kim's Mum always tells you: everything is meant for a reason, even when you don't know why.

I was weary, but I knew that my inner voices were right. If I gave up, I didn't know when or how I would find the courage to try again.

If I was going to go through hell, I was only passing through. I would not purchase a return ticket.

It's OK to Take a Step Back and Find Your Footing

I survived extremely battered, but I managed to still have a pulse. One would think that I would have been ecstatic, right? In reality, I was actually too damaged from the fight to celebrate the victory. Once the physical ordeal had lessened, there was still a feeling of having been turned inside out. I felt like the debris that is left after a tornado or hurricane has decimated a village during a natural disaster.

Yes, I was immensely proud of the victory. It would take a long time to feel anything close to being whole. I didn't share that with anyone. Not because there weren't people who were more than willing to listen and be there for me, I just couldn't put the true emotional cost of the ordeal into words.

Everything seemed to take 100 times the effort that it would normally take. I looked complete on the outside, but the inside was more of a teardown and rebuild. It is entirely possible that the whole thing made me somewhat irrational. You see, I decided that as I was already feeling broken I should try and come off of my other two medications while I was on a roll and get the whole ordeal over and done with. I know, crazy right?

Naturally, I wouldn't stop both of the other ones at the same time. I decided to just follow the same advice that I had been given about methadone. Probably not my smartest move because every drug could be different as far as withdrawal goes. I didn't have the fight in me that I had had with the methadone withdrawal, this was far more civilized though. For one thing, I cut back much more slowly. It wasn't with the same urgency as the methadone. I would make an adjustment and then live with that for a little while, then reduce again and so on. This is not an endorsement that any reader should reduce medications without consulting their doctor. Health-care professionals are the only ones who know each person's individual risks and health needs. **Once again do not try this at home.**

There wasn't the same intensity as far as any side effects this time. It was unpleasant, but these things are never easy. I am extremely glad that I tackled the methadone withdrawal first, otherwise I would have had a rude awakening expecting the methadone to be relatively easy. I wanted to surprise Kim, so I kept it a secret from him. We don't usually keep secrets unless it is about Christmas or birthday gifts. If there is a secret in our household it's for a good cause and something that the person will really love when it comes time for the big reveal. I knew it would blow Kim away if we could put medication behind us once and for all.

The only reason Harley knew of this new self-inflicted challenge was that he was keeping a close watch on my health and if I didn't have the energy to do the exercise, etc., or perhaps something stood out as being out of the ordinary to him, I figured I would nip his concerns in the bud and give him the explanation beforehand. It seemed logical to me that if he knew ahead of time he would tailor my fitness program accordingly.

Harley didn't push me as much physically as he was accustomed to doing while I went through my withdrawal phase. He already knew that my body was encountering enough of a challenge and not to add to it for a while. I never told him what the withdrawal was doing to me physically, at least not in any detail. There were days when going to the gym was nearly impossible, but I went anyway. The gym was the portal to my intended life. I needed to keep that portal open until I was healthy enough to step through it and leave behind my living nightmare once and for all.

During this time Harley focused instead on more gentle pursuits.

One day out of the blue he said to me, "We need to do something about the way that you walk," and motioned me to follow him into the studio space. No one had addressed the way that I walked before. We were alone as he began to demonstrate how to walk properly. I began to laugh.

"OK sure, but how is that different than how I walk?" I questioned. "Well, your walk is more awkward for one thing. It's like this."

With that, he walked the way that I guess I must do. Naturally, I don't go around watching myself walk, so how would I know such things? I would imagine that his depiction of me was pretty accurate, but I can't say for certain. Seeing the two moves it was obvious that my walk was way off, as the two versions looked nothing alike.

"But Harley, you walk like a man so it's nothing like the way a girl walks," I pointed out.

"Hmm, you might have a point."

With that, Harley went into his thinking pose.

As fate would have it, moments later a young woman walked into the room and I could see Harley studying how she was walking with great intensity. She had no idea that he was intending to use the way she walked as a training tool to teach me how it should be done. She had only come in to get some equipment.

Once she left, Harley took a moment to gather his thoughts. "OK try this, then."

With that, he began walking the length of the room. In his demonstration, he absolutely nailed the way that the woman had been walking. I wish I could have filmed his performance because it was priceless.

I couldn't believe that he imitated her walk in order to teach me how to move properly. Fortunately, I was the only witness so Harley's macho image can remain intact. To this day, that is one of my favourite moments of hanging out with him. He was obviously willing to do anything—even risking looking foolish—if it meant it would help me. That told me a lot about how invested he was in getting me better.

Harley has a definite business persona. He can be very

matter of fact, but also has cheerleading and motivating people down to a science. Truth be told, he actually is a bit of a chameleon. When he wants to, he can fit in with the iron-pumping, testosterone-fueled crowd one minute, and then seamlessly join a frustrated senior having difficulty with motion the next. He picks up on what is going on around him and acts accordingly.

It was during the drug withdrawal that I really got to see an entirely softer side to him. Instead of starting our workout right away with an onslaught of exercises, he would sit down beside me, and ask how I was holding up. I had become accustomed to the fact that he was anticipating an answer from me, so I gave him just enough information to answer his questions without going into every minute detail of what I was experiencing. He would make a note in his paperwork each time my medication level changed for later reference should he need it.

Only when he was satisfied that I was feeling up to the task, would he suggest beginning the exercises. Although he always had a long list of things he wanted to accomplish in my hour with him, that was all secondary. Nothing was more important than how I was feeling. For these few months, how I was coping with my withdrawal symptoms determined the direction we would take during our sessions together.

On more than one occasion, he told me that he felt honoured to be part of my journey and I know that he meant it. I appreciated the sentiment. Harley has a hidden soft centre, perhaps I was just seeing his own pilot light shining.

He still had me exercising like crazy. He might have been a little gentler but he certainly wasn't shying away from challenging me, by any stretch of the imagination. It just wasn't as physically hard-core. He was making up for that by making my brain ache.

By the time I conquered my need for medications I was a triumphant battle fatigued warrior princess. In those challenging weeks, I had achieved the impossible and become medication-free. When multiple highly educated medical professionals say that there is nothing that can be done, you tend to believe them, yet here I was achieving something that I had repeatedly been told could not be done.

It was Christmas time when I finally got off of the medications for good. We had gone over to our niece's house for Christmas dinner. It was a lovely small family evening, and after the wonderful turkey dinner with all of the fixings, I told them all that I had managed to stop taking my medications. It was in the early days of that success, but I knew it was safe to share the news with them as there wasn't a hope in hell that I would go back after everything I had just put myself through.

I did say that I was off of the medications using the plural tense. As I had anticipated, Kim explained to everyone that I meant I was off of the methadone. I was beyond excited to be able to correct him. "No, sweetheart, I am now off of all of my medications. Merry Christmas! I've been saving your best Christmas present for last."

It actually took him a few moments to realize exactly what it was that I had just said and what it meant. That was a very emotional Christmas day as we celebrated together. It is a Christmas memory that I will always treasure.

Who would have thought that teaming up with an eager, resourceful, personal trainer, combined with some pretty strong willpower on my part, would mean that we could prove the medical profession wrong? Together, Harley and I had become a mighty dragon-slaying duo.

What completely blows my mind is this: if I was off medication with no difference in my pain levels, had all those toxic concoctions for all of those years been totally unnecessary? If I had just moved my body instead, would it have been possible not to trigger the electric shock onslaught? I will never know the answers for certain, but all I can say is, it gets me thinking.

Being able to be medication-free clearly displays the overwhelming benefit of exercise. I had come from struggling to lift my feet two centimetres from the ground and holding them there, to being medication free, even if it wasn't pain-free yet, Harley had earned my greatest respect and eternal gratitude.

Have I Lost My Mind, or Found it?

To work on my balance and co-ordination, Harley would build an obstacle course that I had to attempt to navigate. First there was a section of square blocks that he would position just the way he wanted them, once in place I had to step through them without falling over. It reminded me of the tires you would see people run through when they are training for football, or doing an obstacle course just on a smaller scale. I would step out of the blocks immediately onto a Bosu, balance there momentarily before transitioning to perhaps a wooden plank to walk along making sure to avoid falling off if at all possible. The final move was up and over a balance board. Once I safely got to the end, I had to go back through it all again to return to the start. The square blocks were always first, but the order of the obstacle course altered depending on what was available or what struck Harley's fancy that day. I never got through one of his obstacle courses without holding on for dear life. Now I think about it, it was very much like the agility courses you see dogs use. I guess all creatures need to be agile.

He always built the course against the wall, and then he would be on the other side of me. That way I could catch myself on the wall or hold onto him as we went along. He stuck to me like glue, and had to be prepared for anything. I was all over the place.

One thing I appreciated was the fact that he didn't stop part-way through and make me begin again. No matter how many times I touched the wall or held onto Harley's arm for balance, we always completed the entire thing and then did it all over again as many times as he wanted.

If the balance work wasn't enough, Harley added a neurological component. He was trying to get my brain to let go of sending the constant pain signals that I was receiving. There isn't one specific exercise that can do that.

The science of neuroplasticity deals with the ability of the brain to form new connections and pathways. It changes how the brain is wired so that over time, the brain alters its patterns of response. That is what Pam was doing during neurological physiotherapy, and what Harley was attempting to do as well. He reasoned that my brain had gotten stuck in a loop, so if he could get my muscles to function properly and the brain to bypass that loop, my pain could potentially go away.

This is a very specialized scientific field. To better understand the topic, I read a couple of books by best-selling author Dr. Norman Doidge: *The Brain That Changes Itself*, and *The Brain's Way of Healing*.

Neuroscience is a fascinating field, but as someone who is not scientifically inclined, the subject was sometimes difficult to comprehend. Nonetheless, both books were worth reading. If you are interested in reading more about neuroplasticity,

I invite you to go to your neighbourhood library or type "books on neuroplasticity" into Google, and you will be presented with large selections of books on the subject.

Neurological exercises are a lot like magic. When you observe a talented magician, you intensely watch to see if you can figure out how the trick is done. The magician can even tell you that they are going to be tricking you, so you are making sure not to let that happen, and yet we are still fooled. It's an optical illusion, you can't see the ball move from one place to another even though it does. You are always left wondering how they did it.

It was the neurosurgeon who told me the brain doesn't take in everything that we see. It takes in a certain amount and then fills in the rest of the picture based on what it assumes that picture should look like. This is what the magician is counting on. Even when a trick is done slowly enough that you think you have seen it all, the magician is successful because of our brain's auto-fill feature.

Harley's neurological exercises made my brain so full that it didn't have time to react in its usual fashion. It had to achieve what I was trying to do in a new way. When you keep forcing the brain to work differently, it eventually lets go of how you have done something all along. Then you are left with how you want the brain to do the task going forward.

Neurological exercise is not one-time work. Once you perfect an exercise, you have to do it over and over again. I can't wake up one morning and decide my brain is going to react differently, it doesn't work like that. Harley and I have been working on my walking, on and off, for years now. When we began, I felt extremely disoriented and slightly nauseous. I thought that I was going to fall over. Holding myself in a corrected posture hurt because my body wasn't used to it.

I could only walk the new way a few minutes at a time. I built up my tolerance by working at it every day. It was only after my brain accepted that this was my natural way to move that we could look at fine-tuning things further. In my case, it took about three years to go from concentrating on every aspect of my movement to walking that way without thinking. Not all brain rewiring takes as long as mine has, but I believe that the delay was because we were trying to change a lifelong condition.

Harley isn't a specialist in neuroplasticity. I don't know if he had tried neuroplasticity principles with any other client before. At first, I wasn't aware of what he was trying to do. With Pam, I knew going in, because her work involved the brain. With Harley, I was just working hard on things that I didn't see other people at the gym doing.

Harley and I never sat down to discuss what we were going to try. We were both just open-minded and willing to try anything. If he read up on anything that he thought could make a difference, it was worth exploring and we would give it a go. He didn't have to tell me what he was up to.

I think that Harley's ability to look at the body in its entirety is what sets him apart from your standard personal trainer. His clients come to him and say that they have an issue in one specific area, but he never simply gives them a set list of exercises to do. He gets busy investigating the cause, which might end up being something you think is completely unrelated. Yes, the more I know Harley, the more he proves to me that he is from another planet.

One day the two of us were talking and Harley said he didn't quite understand why some things that he thought would be easy and straightforward were sometimes the hardest things for him to show me how to do. Yet with far more advanced moves, he is blown away when I pick them up with relative ease.

I explained my take on the situation this way. Since birth, my brain has had faulty wiring. Over time, my body has somehow learned how to adapt in order to do things, but not necessarily using the right brain transmissions or muscle groups to get the job done. That was my simplified version of the neurosurgeon's box analogy. Anytime Harley tried to get me to do something that my brain had already created its own way of doing, it automatically routed through the damaged part of my brain. Whereas for the brand-new stuff that my brain didn't have a pattern for, it created a whole new sequence and stored it in the newly used part of the brain. Then I could call on that newly stored information to reproduce the movement at my request. It's a very unscientific view, but I believe that's what was happening.

One example of the difficulties that we encountered when rewriting a pre-existing movement pattern in my brain would be when Harley would breakdown a move like he had done countless times before. Take a basic step-up exercise for example:

To execute a step up, stand parallel to a step,

1. Place the leg closest to the step onto the step,

2. Bring the other leg up as though you were about to march,

3. Balance with the raised leg up for a moment, and then bring it down.

Harley showed me how to do the step-up properly and I would practice until I got it right. Then he would ask me to do the same move, but change it slightly.

1. Start by crossing over the outside leg, in front of the leg closest to the step,

2. Bring the outside leg onto the step,

3. Bring the other leg from behind, up into the marching position and hold it. Then lower the leg back down again.

In this case, all I was doing was changing the leg I pushed off with. But my brain would not comprehend that simple fact. To me, they were two different exercises that I believe needed to be learned separately. There was no connection between the two.

The same thing would happen to me with different exercises if Harley asked me to change sides and continue on. Not only did I not know how to do that, but my brain would freeze. I suddenly could no longer do the exercise I was just doing moments before, because I had become too confused.

The Pilot Light Effect

It was as though my brain deleted that first file entirely. It wouldn't register that there was any connection at all to my existing move. This was an entirely different matter and my brain would be prepared to get out the excavators in order to create a new neurological path that it was convinced that I needed.

This would end up frustrating us both. Harley would try any way he could think of to get through to me. I would repeat the move as requested only to hear, "No, do it again." Eventually, Harley would move on to something else because we clearly weren't getting anywhere with what he was trying to show me.

Nothing would be gained by making me feel defeated. I think Harley had exhausted all of his usual tricks. He would go home though and research the situation to discover if there was something he was missing, or a different exercise that he could use to bring about the desired result.

I give Harley an A for effort when it comes to the neurological work. I asked him why we didn't just skip that step and simply move on to the next thing. With a wise look, he said that in order to move on to the next thing that he wanted to show me, I needed to be able to do this move first.

Whenever we needed to use my older brain wiring, it was a tough go and could literally take months to master the move. Then one day out of the blue I could move the muscle Harley wanted or perform the movement to his exacting standards. It was hit and miss at first, but we were making progress.

I think it is vitally important to remain open-minded. New techniques, especially in the area of health, are being developed all the time. I wouldn't say I wanted to be a human guinea pig, but if it had no harmful long-term effects, I always agreed to at least try. If what we tried didn't work for me, I always figured that at least Harley might have learned something that could help someone else later.

Sometimes You Aim for the Stars

I have been known to aim high throughout my life. I always shoot for the stars and although they are light years away and out of reach, the view alone has always been worth the effort.

When you are victorious in battle, it is sometimes hard not to let that mess with your head. I was definitely in the outer stratosphere, well beyond cloud nine when it came to how thrilled I was to be off of the pain medications. It took me a long time not to automatically beam every time Harley looked at me after that. I would tell myself that next time he looks in my direction I won't react, just nod. But invariably he would glance over from time to time and the beaming smile instantly materialized into full display for everyone to see.

Now we both knew I had every reason to be beaming and seeing as it was directly related to what he had been able to do for me, it is only obvious that he would be the recipient. No one else at the gym knew.

They just saw this massive smile and probably wondered what the heck was going on.

I've told Harley many times how grateful I am and how much

I appreciate his hard work. Somehow though it isn't really appreciation in the normal sense of the word. I appreciate it when my sister picks up something for me when she is out shopping. I appreciate when Kim has made a nice dinner for us to enjoy together, and I appreciate it when I get to spend time with those that I love. This was none of those things. I was the recipient of abilities that I never dreamt were possible. This young man gave me the gift of a new quality of life, for which I had been searching since I was the uncoordinated four-year-old trying to avoid being hit with a ruler. It was as though all of my Christmases have come at once. Thank you can't begin to cut it.

I am pleased to report that I have since managed to stop automatically beaming when he is in my vicinity, thank goodness, but I think the gratitude will be with me forever.

Once I felt it was safe to let Dr. Welsh know what I had done, I let him in on my secret. I couldn't conceal it from him, he would have been expecting me to obtain repeat prescriptions from him that I did not need. He was amazed at my accomplishment and seemed genuinely pleased for me, but I fully understood if he didn't approve of my methods. He couldn't endorse having his patients take matters into their own hands. It would go against his many years of medical training. He also knew that were it not for a guardian angel looking out for me, things could have taken a life-altering turn for the worse. In hindsight, I would be more cautious now. My strong mindedness would have still wanted me off of the medications, but I would certainly have created more of a safety net.

Now that I have had time to reflect on the matter, I believe that doctors in our current medical system tend to handle acute care, whereas Harley is more of a lifestyle specialist. Both have their unique spots when it comes to health care, there are benefits and room for both to coexist.

In Harley's favour, he has had many hours with me to achieve what we have done. Every one of those hours has been extremely well spent. Whereas with Dr. Welsh the demands for his expertise dictate that he only has a few minutes to assess the situation and take action. It is not an equal playing field by any means

He did say to me on a subsequent visit to his office several months later that he had had no intention of ever taking me off of the pain medications. That took an awful lot for him to admit. I respected that. Even though we might have approached things differently on this one issue, he had worked tirelessly behind the scenes within the medical profession as my advocate trying to get me in to see someone who could help me. He remained a crucial part of my team.

I thought people came off of methadone all of the time. I didn't think that I had achieved anything out of the ordinary. Sometimes, if you don't get the memo that something is next to impossible to achieve, you have a better chance of being triumphant simply because it hasn't occurred to you not to go for what you want.

I frequently compare my health recovery to mountain climbing. It's a monumental task that takes immense dedication as well as physical and mental fortitude. Although I am alone in many ways it takes a team to support the effort. Mountaineers invest in the best equipment available, train hard, and rely heavily on the expertise of people on the expedition with them, I was no different.

You can't summit Mount Everest by thinking that you are done upon arriving at the first base camp. There is literally a mountain of work required in order to reach the peak. I have so many areas of my body in need of a great deal of attention that we could probably work on them for decades to come. Not that the achievement of getting off of pain medications didn't warrant some sort of fanfare. It did. I was simply smart enough to realize that this needed to be only the beginning and not the conclusion of my efforts. We were metaphorically speaking, still at base camp.

Harley told me once that if there was a scale where the start of being fit was at zero, and you went up or down from there as you got fitter, he would put me somewhere around a -10 or -11 if I remember the numbers correctly. Ouch! That stung. I couldn't fault him because he was absolutely right. He just had the guts to tell me things as he saw them. I needed to hear that. It told me loud and clear that there was an awful lot to do. I was a long way from what Harley even considered a starting point. That's one way to be brought back down to earth in a hurry.

The view can be quite inspiring even from base camp, with a buzz in the air. Thoughts begin to wander back to that time where the living room felt miles away. A good day was decent viewing on the television and relief was found in a syringe.

There was no desire to go back there. My pilot light was feeling stronger now than it had in a long time. I could finally take it off of auto-pilot and regain the controls. This felt amazing, even though I was hesitant. I was ready to let the fire build.

As I turned my gaze back towards the mountain standing there in all its splendor, I took a deep breath in and tried to settle my racing heart. This is it... I am going for the summit where the air is thin and the stars abundant. The world of my own creation awaits.

The Fire is Blazing

As wonderful as it is to achieve a level of success, it is unrealistic to believe that you don't go through peaks and valleys. I can't expect every workout to be worthy of fanfare. I put in a lot of hours that no one sees, in order to achieve one small thing. You think that nothing is happening in your body until you suddenly see undeniable proof that what you are doing is creating monumental change.

My own irrefutable proof happened one seemingly ordinary morning quite out of the blue. I woke up feeling really good. That should have been my first clue. That never happened to me. You would think not having stabbing pains would have alerted me that something extraordinary was going on, but it didn't.

I had gone out and done some errands with Kim. It wasn't until much later that afternoon that it dawned on me that I hadn't experienced a stabbing pain since around the same time the previous day. Holy crap! How on earth could I miss that. I had gone 24 hours pain-free. After waiting 12 years, it was unfathomable to me that such an auspicious occasion would pass by almost unnoticed. I could have cried right there on the spot. It was overwhelming, as I hadn't allowed myself to dare to dream that this was even a possibility, never mind being able to experience such a phenomenon for myself. It continues to give me tingles every time I think of it.

The Pilot Light Effect

I could hardly contain my excitement as I ran as quickly as I could to tell Kim the spectacular news. I have committed to memory the look of astonishment on his face. Neither of us could believe what I was saying. We didn't quite know how to react. Of course, we were mentally popping the champagne cork and getting the party streamers out in celebration. Our only hesitancy was the thought that this could be just a fleeting moment. The pain could have gone into hiding temporarily, but if this was a dream then don't wake me up.

Once I had calmed down sufficiently to think straight, my very next task on the agenda was to e-mail Harley and share my tremendous news with him. I have never seen him respond to an e-mail as fast as that one. It might have been the fact that the subject line read YOU ARE A GENIUS that grabbed his attention. At that moment, to me, he was indeed a freaking genius, and I didn't mind telling him so. He was over the moon for me. This was, after all, what we had both been working so hard to achieve for such a long time. He knew the amount of work we had both invested into making this day possible.

It was a peculiar sensation indeed, being pain-free after 12 years of tortured existence. I had forgotten what pain-free living felt like. At first, I thought that I must be in some sort of alternate dimension. I needed to pinch myself to make certain that it was all real. There was a sense of wonder, I felt like a small child discovering that Santa had left gifts for everyone under the twinkling Christmas tree. I wouldn't describe myself as radiant, but I was radiating that day. My body was awash with emotion.

Although the customary pain had vanished, I was still getting the sensation of the pain going through the motions of building towards its customary crescendo, and just at the apex, as I prepared for the jolt the nerves brushed by one another without making contact. The bolt never materialized. For the first little while, I would think to myself that I had escaped that particular shock, but surely the next one would be a doozie. My entire body was on high alert, waiting for something to happen.

That first night, I was still so beside myself with pure joy, but I was scared to let myself sleep. I didn't want to wake up the next day with the pain back in full force. I believed the longer I was awake the less chance there was that the pain could sneak back.

Kim was sound asleep beside me. I had no one to talk to, so I put some headphones on to listen to some music and reflect upon the thrill of the day. I didn't sleep more than two or three hours during that entire time, because I was too busy savouring every second of it. What sleep I did get that night was from sheer exhaustion.

The pain managed to stay away for close to 36 hours before returning with full force. That was a blow, but it wasn't as though I didn't expect it. To be honest being pain-free had lasted much longer than I thought it would.

I should have been crestfallen when the pain reappeared, but I wasn't. Sure, I was disappointed, but I started to look at the whole thing with more of a scientific experiment rather than my customary emotional approach. I was paying extra close attention to what my nerves were doing to see if I could figure out the difference between what I felt when the nerves missed each other and when they connected, other than the obvious statement that one hurts and one doesn't. Not allowing myself to be discouraged, I used it as even more incentive to keep going. If it happened once, it can happen again.

The latest revelation added fuel to my fire. Working out with Harley and successes such as this was a constant source of inspiration. My self-confidence skyrocketed, and I was feeling unstoppable. This was the power surge my pilot light had been hoping for. The fact that my light now glowed was undeniable. I wondered what else I was capable of doing? What if I could actually get well. I mean being on the positive side of Harley's scale definition of well. What would that feel like?

I decided not to alter anything drastically, at least not for the moment. I needed time to take it all in and decipher how I could consistently get the zap to fail. My mission became focused on observing how my body moved to look for subtle changes and anything else that I could notice.

I had never paid so much attention to my own body. I was having a crash course on what everyone assumes should be second nature. The signs were all there as to what part of my body was working and what wasn't. The failure on my part was my inability to interpret my own body language. It could be said that I was so out of sync that it had taken the shock waves for me to notice, even then these alarm bells fell on deaf ears until now.

I was convinced that it was a combination of both my brain and my body, and somewhere between the two was my get-out-of-jail-free card. My brain had to somehow stop creating the neurological impulse and my body had to let go of its lifelong propensity to twist my muscles into massive knots rendering them useless. In my own fashion, I understood on a very elementary level what needed to happen.

I hadn't the first clue how that was going to be accomplished, so I did what anyone in my position would have done. I passed the task over to Harley. He might not have figured it out entirely either, but if anyone could solve the puzzle, my bet was on him.

This is where having other people to turn to for guidance was a gift. There is a huge difference between contributing towards an objective and being dictated to. I had a voice, this was my life.

Harley knew that his customized exercise regime, if done properly and frequently, over time would lead to better balance, strength, and a multitude of other health benefits. There was no need to change anything on that score. What piqued his interest was what could be accomplished through increased emphasis on my neurological challenges.

The Million Piece Jigsaw Puzzle

Every now and again, I get it into my head to try something that I haven't been able to do for a long time just to see if I can do it. It is always such a nice surprise when an ability returns. It was a cause for celebration when I regained the ability to step off of a curb. Being able to do that was so liberating, any anxiety I would customarily feel when approaching a curb now has evaporated.

You don't notice the exact moment that your body can no longer perform a specific function until you go to do it and discover that the ability has gone. I have now discovered that it is the exact same thing in reverse when you get an ability back. The abilities don't come back in any logical order. It's all quite random and most certainly not in order of importance. That doesn't really matter though. I just put out my welcome back banner.

When you are trying to put your health back together, it's very much like doing a million-piece jigsaw puzzle, where all the puzzle pieces are tiny, yet essential. It was around the five-year mark of working with Harley that I discovered that I now have the ability to go backward automatically.

Before, stepping backwards took tons of concentration, was

very awkward and unstable.

I hadn't even realized that my brain had created a compensatory pattern. Instead of going backward, I just automatically turned around and always faced forward. I actually wasn't aware that my reverse capability was missing.

The brain must know that the new ability is ready to be used somehow though, because all on its own, it had stopped me turning around automatically, and started directing me to go backward normally.

Each time that I learned a new ability, Harley went into overdrive. The reason for that was critically important. He wanted to make certain that while the brain is accepting the fact that I could now do this new task, it wasn't learning how to do the movement improperly. He called that neurological mapping. It makes sense if you stop to think about it.

If we look upon the brain as a human supercomputer, when you program a function into a computer, you make certain the data is pristine, that way, each time you retrieve that file, you perform that function perfectly. It is the same thing when neurologically mapping. We are just making sure that my brain has retained all the updates and goes to my new ability file rather than my old one.

Most of my own original movement patterns have been in some way neurologically corrupted. I have had decades of doing things incorrectly. One by one, we painstakingly correct them. It's an arduous task, but so rewarding when I do a movement correctly that I haven't been able to do before.

We have all heard the saying, "You can't teach an old dog new tricks." That may or may not be true of the canine kingdom, but I am living proof that that saying doesn't apply to humans.

As a neurological exercise, Harley decided to show me some stick work. He explained to me that he would move towards me very slowly with a long wooden pole. My only job was to face him and avoid the pole. It should be simple right? True to form, for me, it wasn't. Each time he approached me, I had no idea what way I needed to move in order to avoid the pole. I would just freeze on the spot. Most of the time I went in the wrong direction entirely. Each time that happened, Harley would pause and indicate which way I should be going. He would then patiently wait for me to avoid the pole. I didn't have a headache after that exercise, I had a full-on brain ache.

We had been at this for quite a while and have managed to teach my brain to react to an object coming towards me. Even if Harley came at me at a faster pace, my brain knew which way my body needed to go. He taught me to react. I do get it wrong sometimes, but it is nothing like how I used to be. When I get it wrong, I don't just stand there in a fog as before. Instead, my brain realizes that I have made an error and attempts to correct it. At least now I recognize it as an error.

We are currently working on defensive moves, as well as how to initiate, anticipate and react to what is around me. When I eventually get that down, Harley will inevitably come up with a new neurological challenge for us to work on. I don't tell people that I can't do something unless I am out of options, and one day I ran out of options when I was with Harley. He made me do an exercise with a weighted ball. If I am not mistaken, the exercise consisted of me doing a squat while holding onto the ball, then raising up, tossing the ball in the air, catching it and then repeating the two moves until he told me to stop.

At the risk of appearing stupid, I had to tell him that I couldn't catch. No one wants to admit that they can't catch something when they are nearly 60 years old. It's like not being able to ride a bicycle or swim, I didn't want to let the world in on my secrets. Sure, I would catch the odd ball or two growing up, that's the law of averages, isn't it? The catches were very few and far between. As a rule, playing catch was more a game of watching the ball drop and then retrieving it. It wasn't a lot of fun.

I was equally as bad at throwing the ball back. It traveled wherever it felt like and seldom where I thought that I sent it. Playing catch with me was a dangerous sport indeed. Now here Harley was, wanting me to toss a weighted ball. All I could think was that I was going to end up with broken toes.

As soon as I confessed to Harley that I couldn't catch, he said, "But a girl needs to know how to catch. Follow me."

"Harley, I have managed without being able to catch so far, I just need you to stop giving me an exercise that involves catching weighted balls, that's all."

I couldn't say any more to him because he was already

several strides ahead of me walking towards the studio space. He had abandoned what we were doing at the time and was now on a mission to show me how to catch. There was no point protesting, I followed him into the vacant room where we were out of the way and couldn't hurt anyone.

He grabbed a Pilates ball, as he went past the equipment area and stood facing me.

"You really think you can teach me to catch? Good luck with that because I don't think it can be done," I said with conviction.

"Oh! You think so, do you?"

"Let's see which one of us is right. Challenge accepted," he said with a gleeful twinkle in his eyes.

Oh my God what have I done? I had seen that look before, and it always involved tons of work.

We stood closely together facing one another.

"OK Maria, we are going to just start with me throwing the ball to you slowly. Cup your hands together like so, and let me worry about getting the ball to you. You just keep your hands together."

I was too busy laughing to respond to him.

I watched as he threw the ball to me, and it landed into my hands just as he said it would.

"I didn't really do anything, Harley. I only caught it because you threw it directly into my hands."

"True, but you didn't let the ball pass through your fingers, so therefore you caught it. Well done."

"Now throw the ball back to me."

I made a feeble attempt to toss the ball back to him, which he needed to retrieve.

"Now I am going to try throwing to you again, just keep your hands ready."

My laughter was beginning to subside, so I was better able to focus with the next toss. Once again it landed perfectly, exactly where Harley had aimed it. This was clearly due to Harley's ability to throw correctly rather than any newly found aptitude on my part to catch.

Over the next few minutes, he moved further away from me or changed the angle of the throw. Sure, quite a few balls were dropped, but I managed to catch more balls in that 10 minutes than all the previous catches I had ever made before.

"I'll be damned. I might not be any good at it, but I think you might have just taught me the very basics of catch and throw, that's incredible. You win."

Harley smiled brightly. "I knew I'd win, all we need to do now is work on it, that is going to be our new exercise."

"That's impressive, wait until I get home and tell Kim, he's not going to believe it. Thanks for that."

I gave Harley a big hug in appreciation of his efforts.

Sometimes I wonder if my body became so accustomed to Harley making me do something new, that it saw him coming and just surrendered saying, *OK, just do what he says and no one needs to get hurt.* There is also a possibility that he has trained to be a magician. If neither of these things was true, then we somehow transformed my brain.

When people see Harley coming at me with a stick or tossing a ball at me, they can be excused for thinking that it doesn't appear to look like exercise. We look as though we are playing when in actuality, it is a great deal of work. It's a challenging exercise for me. I can physically feel my brain trying to work. It is exhausting. When it comes to brain exercising, I can only take a few minutes at a time. My brain gets overloaded and doesn't know how to reply to the stimulation.

A case in point was the occasion when my brain had so much going on simultaneously that my feet didn't go in the direction I intended them to go and I simply fell. Harley and I were at the gym, working on my stick work when the fall happened. It was unlike any fall I had ever experienced before. Customarily once a fall began, I had no concept of how to save myself from falling or minimize the impact. I would go down with an almighty thud and then assess the damage.

I fell two or three times a year during my descent years, out of the blue I would find myself on the ground in a heap. Thankfully, I didn't sustain any injuries when I fell which was sheer luck. This was the only time I have fallen since teaming up with Harley. I was perfectly fine, it was only my brain having a glitch. The reason it happened wasn't stupidity on my part or negligence on Harley's. It was simply a circuit overload. Neither of us knew my brain's simultaneous stimuli capacity.

My brain doesn't make changes unless it sees no other option, so it was quite normal to be doing more than one thing concurrently. If you try to pat your head while rubbing your belly, you would begin to understand how difficult it is to do two neurological challenges at the same time. Now that we have a better understanding of my stimuli limits, Harley has been very careful about how much we try to get the brain to do at any given time. It is all a learning curve as we work to reconstruct my puzzle pieces.

It's only someone like me who would be excited by a fall. That's because, this time, the fall felt as though it was happening in super slow motion, my brain was trying to think of an appropriate action to take. Although I was unsuccessful in saving myself, it was the first time my brain has ever reacted to a fall, which made me very happy.

Although I thought I was in slow motion, according to Harley my fall was too quick for him to be able to prevent it. We were both surprised that it happened, but as I was fine, we carried on.

With any million-piece jigsaw puzzle, you have to tackle it a bit at a time in sections. There is no way that you can power through and get the puzzle completed quickly. Much like when you gather all of the edge pieces together or the sky section, all the remaining pieces of the puzzle remain in the box until it is their turn to be placed.

Harley and I have had to do that as well. For me, the first priority was pain management and then medication removal. The only way to achieve that was to start getting the muscles active and participating. There are estimated to be 650 named skeletal muscles in the human body. Getting that many muscles to work simultaneously, Harley had to become a bit of a movement mechanic.

The skeletal muscles are the ones that enable movement, those are the ones that have been our biggest focus. You can't ignore the cardiac muscles, so they went on our priority list as well. Any muscle that is capable of working without conscious awareness though, we don't spend too much time worrying about. Harley is kept busy working the different muscle groups and seems to cycle through most areas of concern on a regular basis.

When you are going into such fine detail, things take time. Sometimes it can feel like we are trying to spin plates. We get one area working, and then something else stops spinning. We rush to that area just in time to get the spin back under control, then try to get another muscle or two spinning along.

How does a simple gym girl make sense of it all? As things got better my excess weight started to disappear, and my focus turned to establishing better eating habits. Life-long habits are hard to change. I have periods where I eat much better and then things slide a little. I tend to be an emotional eater, so I try to avoid things that will cause me to turn to food for comfort.

When I was the human exemplification of a sedentary rock, I wouldn't really eat that much. If the food was not within arm's reach, it would take something extra special to make me get up and shuffle towards the kitchen. Don't forget I had to consider that there was always a return trip to the couch involved in my "Is it worth it?" calculations.

Check any dictionary and the definition of diet would be: limiting food to improve your physical condition and lose weight. I figured if I was offered a sweet treat I should just enjoy it, I even deserved it, because there wasn't much to enjoy going on in my world. The problem with that is, I wasn't doing anything to burn it off. The calories would just settle in with all the other fat and take up residence. Even if I ate 500 calories a day, which is not a lot, how many calories can a person burn on an average day just sitting? I have no idea, but it can't be that much. Interestingly Harley doesn't refer to it as weight loss. He calls it fat loss. I guess you could lose water or muscle weight if it comes to that, and have technically lost weight, but he said we should be looking for ways to achieve fat loss instead.

Am I the only one on the planet that has never given a moment's thought to the fact that a person actually burns more calories just from choosing to stand up rather than sit down? I wasn't kidding when I said that I had a lot to learn. I am learning new things all the time, it never stops.

I am not actually on a diet. I didn't think to myself that come Monday morning I would give up everything but fruits and vegetables. It's the funniest thing, my body just decided it didn't want what I used to crave, with no coaxing from me.

The Pilot Light Effect

I remember one day quite clearly. I was cooking meat for dinner, and suddenly thought, "This is gross." I had always been a carnivore, so the fact that cooking meat was turning me off wasn't supposed to happen.

I am not a full-blown vegetarian. My body just works fine without meat. I love my fruit and veggies, there are the rare occasions that I have a small amount of flesh though. When I do, I try to eat every morsel and give thanks to the poor animal I am about to consume. I aim to be more conscientious and evolve; I am a work in progress.

The same goes with dairy. The milk that I used to use in a week would now last me anywhere up to two months depending on my mood. My downfall is a wonderful cup of piping hot black tea, complete with a splash of milk being an essential ingredient. I do switch it up with green and fruit teas often, but anyone who knows me well knows I won't be giving up my tea in this lifetime.

What few food vices I enjoy now, I try to keep in moderation. The occasional flare-ups usually correspond to special occasions like Christmas and birthdays, or because it has been so long since I have had a treat that I have begun to worry that I might forget what it tastes like unless I sample it again. That is, unless I let boredom in, then all bets are off.

Our grocery shopping takes place primarily along the outside of the store. Although I have been known to detour down a junk food aisle a time or two, I am only human. The problem with standing in the junk food aisle is that invariably Harley will pop into my head saying, "If you buy it, you will eat it." I hate when that happens, he has given me a food conscience. It's the strangest thing but he never pops into my head when I am looking to buy tomatoes or bananas; it's only when I am drawn to junk food.

Those clothes we all have hidden away at the back of the closet waiting until we get skinnier, started to fit and actually got too big on occasion. Hallelujah! One of my very favourite things to do is periodically go through my clothes and donate all the things I have shrunk out of.

From time to time, I will calculate how long I would have to work out in order to burn off the treat that I want to consume, but it isn't my usual modus operandi. It is always longer than everyone thinks to burn off those pesky calories. It might sound like a delightful idea to grab a coffee and muffin after the gym, but depending on the type of muffin and if the coffee is black rather than of the specialty variety, you could actually consume many times more calories than the ones you just burned off. Life just isn't fair, is it!

I had never really paid attention to my body before, we just sort of hung out together. If my body were writing this book rather than me, it would tell you how mean and neglectful I was, and it would be right. It literally wasn't until there were no other options, that I started to pay attention to it. My body was just like me as a child waiting until the bitter end to be chosen for the team. I owe my body the biggest apology known to man.

A Different Approach

Even though we had been making strides with the neurological pain, there were times when I would experience pain that had nothing to do with my brain. There is a distinct difference between how the pain is felt depending on its origin.

I have become an expert when it comes to pain. Pain that was neurologically based always created a lightning storm of electrical shocks. It was the breath-stealing-cry-out-loud pain that ripped through me without warning. This type of pain had a mind of its own. It defied conventional medical wisdom and did not respond completely to prescribed medications.

When my pain was due to something like pulling a muscle or twisting an ankle, I would get much less severe, more manageable pain. There are no electric shocks to contend with, and traditional fixes such as icing the area or taking an over-the-counter pain reliever usually did the trick. They are both painful experiences, but how I deal with them is completely different.

Harley worked diligently to keep me pain-free, but sometimes when he was not around, I would somehow hurt myself. It always turns out to be operator error on my part, but one way or another, I have to deal with the issue.

On this one occasion, I had been having pain for a few days

that had really grabbed my attention. It wasn't an electric shock so I immediately knew it had a more natural cause. That in itself was good because there are far more options available to me if it isn't neurologically linked.

This pain was somewhere new, at the back of my damaged knee. I am quite accustomed to different pings and pangs coming from that knee from time to time. This wasn't ordinary, in the decades that I have been dealing with this. The back of my knee had always managed to avoid agitation.

The pain was sharp, demanding, and lingering. I did the usual stuff that I do whenever that happens: apply ice, elevate my leg, and take an anti-inflammatory. This time, I got nowhere.

I thought about all the things I had done over the previous few days that might have caused it and was confident that no one particular thing was to blame.

Previously, I would have stayed home and vegetated on the couch, either listening to music or mindlessly watching the television, firmly believing that a few days' rest would absolutely take care of it. The new, slightly wiser me, knew this was exactly the time to avoid the couch, get to the gym, and check-in with Harley. He is, after all, my man with a plan.

He was very quick to agree that my right leg had become very tense. I knew that already because there would be no other reason for it to be hurting me. He began doing some gentle manipulation to the area in question, I could tell when he hit the bullseye as I wanted to scream. After a few unpleasant minutes though I could feel a sense of relief. The rogue muscle was about to surrender. Harley was laser-focused on the task of getting things to return to normal function. Once the correct muscle took on the workload, my pain dissipated, and the muscle resumed its regular duties. It was only once Harley was satisfied that he had achieved what he had set out to accomplish did we return to our usual gym routines. The problem never came back. Those few minutes were all it took to correct the issue. It would have taken weeks had I remained on the couch.

To date, even though I have undoubtedly frustrated Harley on occasion, the frustration traces back to the fact that there seems to be no physical impairment that could satisfactorily explain preventing me from doing any of his exercises, and yet some moves refuse to materialize.

My lats in particular were ridiculously slow. A sloth had nothing on my lats. We worked on getting those working for months. Harley tried every combination of exercises he could think of, even faking it until you could make it produced nothing. So what was I missing? My mind was present, my brain knew the move, and my body made the motion. What more could anyone want? The exercise was becoming futile. Was coming to the gym a waste of time? I was more mildly frustrated, but the scales were about to tip if something didn't happen.

Instinctively, I started back at the very beginning, like those times when you need to retrace your steps while looking for some misplaced treasure, only to discover it right back where you started.

What do you know, suddenly the muscle fired like a fine sports car ready for action. What the heck just happened? Why didn't it do that in the first place?

I learned that it isn't about doing the same things over and over again, to no one's satisfaction. It is about stripping things down and starting from the very beginning. I need my mind, body, and spirit harmoniously committed to each other. When one checks out, nothing happens. It's like trying to get the internet to work without a wifi signal, nothing gets accomplished. It is easy to keep repeating how we do things because it has worked in the past. It takes courage to take things down to the foundation, look at the situation with fresh eyes, and begin again.

The Calf Intervention

My calves have been a knotted mass as far back as I can remember. Like the feet, they also have been nearly impossible to touch. Putting it simply, from the hips down, I am a knotted dysfunctional mess. Thank goodness Harley thrives on challenges. This issue wasn't accident-related, it seemed however that my physical challenges and neurological issues converged to do battle and that battlefield was my calves. The two had somehow intertwined.

The calves had always felt incredibly heavy, as though I am constantly carrying around leaded weights wherever I go. There is no natural lightness or grace to the way that I move, prevented by those lead weights. I am an elephant in human form—and funny enough, a baby elephant is also called a calf.

Although I was thrilled that there has been a huge improvement in my walking since Harley recreated my gait, the calves continued to feel as though I am being stretched so tightly that I was about to snap.

Harley tried manual manipulation on my calves and, oh my God, I had never felt anything like it—even though I claim to be a pain tolerance professional. Nerve conduction tests made my nerves convulse, but the calf stimulation caused a pain that felt as though it was coming from inner earth.

Because the gym is a public place, I couldn't let out any screams. It took everything I had to contain the cries. Even with my best effort, there were more than a few groans each time we dealt with the calves. Harley would try to get me to relax, but when it came to my calves, he didn't stand a hope in hell's chance that I could meditate my way through it all.

Naturally, if you are in the fitness business, the last thing that you want to do is cause a client pain. My body language and facial expression clearly indicated that calf manipulation was something I was not particularly thrilled about. I am sure Harley wondered whether to stop or continue on for my better good.

He said "Maria, I am only pressing ever so lightly," he applied the same force to my arm and I could barely feel it at all. I am certain that he was telling me the truth, but from where I was standing, the two felt as different as night and day.

When he started this practice, I was left with big multi-coloured bruises all over my calves. They would last for days, and you could tell exactly where his fingers had been. That is why I ended up calling the process "fingerprinting" rather than calf manipulation, as it seemed more appropriate. When we began, we had to keep the time we spent working on fingerprinting to no more than 15 minutes. I couldn't have stood it for a moment longer.

In Harley's defence, I have always bruised easily. It really was unavoidable. I wasn't the slightest bit alarmed when the bruises materialized, although I did use it to tease Him that

I now had physical proof of how mean he was, and that maybe he should consider changing his name from Harley to Harshly. The man tolerated a lot of teasing from me. I switched from wearing shorts to workout pants to hide the bruising so that no one could see that my legs were banged up and ask questions.

I can't say that I have ever looked forward to a deep tissue calf massage, I would let him do it simply because it needed to be done. It was a love-hate relationship. I loved the thought of my calves eventually working, but hated the convoluted route we had to take to get there. I would think of how challenging it is to untangle the twisted Christmas tree lights and imagine that that was what Harley was doing to my calves. It seemed only fair to give him the time it takes to get the job done properly, but at the same time, I wished he would hurry up.

Even months later, no matter what Harley tried, he couldn't distinguish a hint of a calf muscle. He had sent out many search parties and came back empty-handed. The instant bruising phase eventually subsided allowing me to wear shorts if I wanted to, alas, that seemed to me to be our only sign of progress. He had countless exercises for just about everything imaginable, but he was dangerously close to exhausting the list of calf exercises he knew trying to help me.

Because I have nothing to compare it to, I don't know how my calves are any different than those of anyone else. I emailed Harley, asking him to explain the differences to me, and he replied by providing me with some notes from my client file:

In my work things often suddenly jump out at me; I'll notice something I didn't notice before, and on this day, it was Maria's calves. Maria's calves were normal size, so my attention had not been drawn to them by any obvious sign until this moment. Calf muscles are integral to balance and ambulation, and since Maria had some challenges with both, I decided to check calf muscle function. The calves looked normal size, yet it was only the surface tissue bulk that was normal. The muscles underneath were thin and soft and buried deep within the surface tissues. I was determined to massage the calf muscles to improve function. There was barely anything to massage! It hit me then, how bio-mechanically challenging life must have been all of her life. When the calves don't work, life is like balancing on stilts.

I massaged and worked Maria's calves for many weeks. Her lower legs were soft and delicate, consisting mostly of tender skin and soft subcutaneous tissues that acquiesced easily to my manual solicitations. The calf muscle was barely discernible from the surrounding tissues, but I could feel the soft ropes.

These soft ropes were very reluctant to produce contractile force. They did not, seemingly could not work. I tried everything: calf raises, standing calf raises, manual resistance, you name it. At a physiological loss, I suggested Maria try some deep meditation to connect mindfully to those long forgotten, underdeveloped baby calf muscles.

In other words, my calves were like the tangled strand of Christmas tree lights. If every other effort was failing me, we were going to need to resort to what could only be described as a calf intervention. Now I truly have heard of everything!

I went home, and over the next few weeks, I would imagine the calves working properly as Harley requested. I would report back in from time to time, but it was a painfully slow process with not much going on. I wondered if Harley couldn't find a functioning calf muscle, I obviously don't have one, and likely never did. If I have never had a functioning calf muscle, how could I know what it is supposed to feel like when it shows up? This was making it a challenge to do the visual imaging. This was well beyond the physical act of doing a deadlift or sit-ups. Now we were playing a different kind of mind game.

I think we must have reached Harley's last idea on the matter in order for him to have mentioned trying visualization. I thought of nothing else other than what I could only imagine a functioning calf muscle would feel like. My mind was once again as empty as an amusement park during a hurricane. I was only thinking of the task at hand and the connection that had been requested. Repeatedly, I tried in vain, there was nothing.

I gave it my best effort to do the assignment. It was pretty vague though. Just imagine your calves working and it would somehow happen. It isn't as though I could make a wish and my fairy Godmother would wave a magic wand, and presto, perfectly functioning calves would materialize. I wasn't having much luck. The whole thing was frankly doing my head in.

I would find a quiet corner at home, usually on the bed or my exercise mat, and try to block out all other thoughts from my mind. My levels of success varied greatly, everything had to be just right in order for my thoughts not to drift towards some household chore that needed to be completed, or what's in the house for dinner. There always seemed to be something else that I would rather be thinking about than my imaginary calf muscles.

It's funny the places your mind goes when it is left to its own devices. I would create random thoughts of being able to do all kinds of physical things once my calves were functioning properly. I would think back to Harley's description of living life on stilts and think, wow! Walking on stilts is a very specialized talent. It's a cool party trick, but certainly not something you want to be doing all of the time. How do I learn to get off of the stilts and walk normally?

With that in mind, I changed what I was usually concentrating on when I let myself imagine. Instead, I simply thought about being off of stilts, so that my mind could remain focused. Once things went out of focus, that was it for the day. Walking without stilts was way easier to think about than something that, for me, never existed.

Each time I managed to achieve some level of success with visualization, my imagination would build on what I had already created. Like a soap opera, the story evolved every time that I tuned in for the next episode.

Although I attempted to have my thoughts revolve around calf muscles, it is a pretty mundane subject and something that I was never going to have any true interest in.

Invariably the visual content moved away from stilts and turned to mighty confrontations. The fight-to-the-death kind of clashes. I could only make sense of it by comparing it to the conflicts I had encountered trying to regain my health. Why else would my mind keep taking me to scenes involving a battlefield?

I was on the verge of waving the white flag of surrender. I decided that I was going to give it just one more attempt to be done with it once and for all; it had all been too much effort for what I was getting out of it. Harley would just have to accept defeat on this one and come up with a different plan of attack.

Sure enough, thoughts of happily moving calves did not stick around for long. Instead, I found myself deep in the forest alone. All around me were these dark shape-shifting creatures. I tried to scream, yet there was no sound. These creatures were communicating among themselves and, although I didn't speak their language, mysteriously I could understand what they were saying. I don't watch or read science fiction, so it fascinated me that my mind was able to create such a sci-fi-like setting.

The creatures were speaking about owning me and that I needed to prepare for combat. In the visualization, I was sobbing uncontrollably but only on the inside. I could not let them see the weakness. The shape-shifters were becoming increasingly stronger; no matter what I did they did not retreat.

When the danger was at its most intense and we prepared for the final death scene. Instead of confronting them as would be expected. I found myself shutting my eyes. Who in their right mind would shut their eyes when they are in imminent danger? I couldn't bring myself to harm the creatures even though they appeared to be quite capable of killing me. When I opened my eyes again the shapeshifters had vanished. Where did they go? What the hell just happened? I frantically searched for them but they had disappeared just as mysteriously as they had arrived. The battle was over and the danger had passed.

In the final scene, I was standing in a field while being told that I had taken on every challenge with dignity, grace, and never gave up believing that this day would happen. For that, I would be rewarded. I was assured that although the work continued, the storm had finally ended. I turned to walk away and discovered a familiar figure in the distance coming to take me home.

On the surface, this might appear to be nothing more than a vivid dream or some mental psychedelic trip. A case could be made either way. It felt alarmingly real to me at that moment. I hadn't taken anything psychedelic and I wasn't asleep or dreaming. When you go through something as horrific as my years of pain have been, it isn't just your body that takes a hit. Your mind can become collateral damage. When your body deteriorates, the mind is on hyper alert, constantly looking for a safe escape route. That response is only meant to be sustained for short periods of time. It's like our fight-or-flight reflex. When you rely on that instinct continually over time, its ability to cope is deteriorated.

Now if we were to look at the body as one self-contained unit—body, mind, and spirit—that changes things. We are no longer a multitude of body parts all harmoniously coexisting. We are one singular perfectly functioning human being.

Within a few weeks of that final visualization, I was doing some seated calf raises, when the seemingly impossible happened. As usual Harley was checking for signs of life in my calf muscles. I didn't give it any thought because it was just routine, he always checks whenever he happens to be working on any one particular muscle group. This time though he got quite the shock when he unearthed the slightest hint of a baby calf muscle attempting to function. We were both astonished. We were in simultaneous silence as we took in the magnitude of the moment. Had the visualization exercise coaxed the muscle into revealing itself? Was it mind over matter that had proven to be the missing component all along? This poor little muscle had never in my life been used before. I was witnessing muscle birth. It was certainly something a person usually doesn't get to experience at my age.

A simple calf visualization exercise was all that was asked for. How it took on a life of its own, I truly do not know. That exercise was every bit as difficult as any of the other ones I have been given. After that experience I announced to Harley that he should come with a warning label. He laughed. The question remains: was I actually kidding?

Of all the many areas we have tackled together, as far as I

am concerned, the calves have easily been the most elusive. Most things have shown progress relatively quickly, but the calves remain a true hurdle to this very day. We were making real headway with deep tissue massage of the calves, but it has to be consistently worked upon. If we miss even a short period of time, my calves revert back to being tangled Christmas tree lights despite all of Harley's valiant efforts.

My calves were the best that they had ever been immediately prior to the outbreak of the COVID pandemic. The global shutdown took every advancement we had made away from me. I did not have access to the gym for months. There was no way to spend time with Harley, and even if there could have been some way to make that happen, he wouldn't have been able to manipulate my calves due to the accepted physical distancing requirements.

I have tried rolling my calves with a foam roller thinking it might help a little, but the calves returned to feeling heavy and tight. I have no idea when we will be able to tackle the calves again the way that we had been doing. My only hope is that once my calves are on Harley's radar again, my body will somehow remember where we had left off and allow me to continue. I think that might be wishful thinking on my part. One thing is for certain Harley will have his work cut out for him, and it will probably be a good idea if I were to wear long pants just in case the bruising comes back.

Reverse Aging

Age is just a number. There are seniors who are fit and young, and old, unfit youngsters as well. Wherever we end up on any fitness scale, we need to take into account lifestyle, amount of exercise, mental well-being, and even socio-economic backgrounds. Every lifestyle choice we make, every setback we encounter, even the comfort foods we turn to, all contribute to our ability to age well. Physically if you can do things now that you couldn't do as a youngster, that to me, is a perfect example of reverse aging.

I was already old when I was in my twenties—talk about having a misspent youth. Now that I feel that I am getting younger, I am experiencing a taste of what it would be like to have a do-over, and I like it. My walker and assorted medical devices are sitting in our storage room collecting dust. Just the other day we were walking through our provincial museum, and one display had a cobblestone street. Although things were uneven underfoot, I navigated through the display well. I wouldn't have been able to do that a few years ago, when my body was older.

Reverse aging puts a spring in your step. Just because I can't deadlift 100 pounds or do a one-armed pull-up doesn't matter. They aren't failures, I look at them as my future successes. I would like to have the upper body strength to be able to pull myself up if I fall overboard somewhere. I also want to be able to go up and down a flight of stairs without holding on. It's always good to have goals, whether you are aging in reverse or not. I have a wish list, and I bet you have one too. There is scientific proof that exercise promotes reverse aging, so maybe exercise is the elusive fountain of youth that everyone is searching for. I watched a program not too long ago about the difference between our chronological age and our biological age, or our calendar age versus the age at which our body performs.

They tested several people of various ages and fitness levels that range from moderately active to sedentary, and were then able to determine their biological age. When they compared the results, it was astonishing.

Without exception, everyone's biological age was much higher—even decades higher than their birth age. Next, they put each of the participants on a medically supervised exercise program based solely on what they were able to do. They didn't send in teams of Harley clones; each person was free to do exactly what they wanted. If they preferred to put in minimal effort or carry on how they had been doing, there were no repercussions.

The team reconvened twelve weeks later and repeated the original testing. This time the results were substantially different. Every one of them had become younger—years younger—biologically speaking. No wonder I feel that I am reverse aging, it's because I am. That explains why I felt so old before too, the fact is, biologically speaking I was. The question is: how old will you biologically be 12 weeks from now?

The Pilot Light Effect

We are always shocked when we hear of someone young dying, it's not supposed to happen that way. It makes me wonder if they might have only been young in the chronological sense. Biologically speaking they died at a ripe old age of natural causes. Yikes!

You might think that by now my Harley Knows Best List is a mile long. I am not going to lie, it is a few pages, and I am fine with that. Some of the exercises have just become second nature and I don't have to go all the way to the gym to do them. I can do some pretty fancy balance moves, while I am standing at the sink waiting for the kettle to boil.

One of the biggest measures of success is being able to translate whatever you want to learn into your daily life. I don't have to be in a gym to be mindful that I am breathing properly. I can work on exercises to strengthen my calves waiting for my bus to come.

Over time, I have gotten some pieces of workout equipment to use at home. During the pandemic, it became very hard to buy equipment, supplies have been low, and the demand was high. I have recently been able to buy some lighter kettlebells. As my capability increases, I will order the next weight up.

It's not the length of your own personal Harley Knows Best List that matters, but rather doing the things that are on it, to the best of your ability on any given day. By doing that, over time, you correct the imbalances your body has created. That makes all of us less unstable on our feet, once we are able to do that an entirely new world of possibilities becomes available to us. Now if that isn't worth turning a few pages over on my Harley Knows Best List each day, then I don't know what is. After all, life is not a spectator sport we all want to be able to get in the game

I only recently got up the nerve to ask Harley where he would put me on his personal fitness scale now. I was at -11 when I started, so I thought I was being conservative when I estimated that I would be a four or five by now. Harley didn't take long to give me his answer. He seemed quite pleased with his decision when he announced that he would put me as a solid two.

It's true that I am thankful to be on the positive side of the equation, but I didn't think I would be quite that low, but he has to take into consideration all of the things that I still don't know how to do. He has a mental list of what a fit person should be capable of doing. I can tick more boxes than I ever have, but there are still tons of boxes needing to be checked off. We should be able to get them all done before I reverse age back to becoming a teenager again.

With COVID and the limited gym access that is available, I lost a little bit of my overall fitness, but some areas have still continued to get better—and my balance is one of those. I plan to be first in line to renew my full gym membership once I can, and then my calves better be ready because fingerprinting will be making a comeback.

Part Three

creating an inferno

Starting at the Beginning

Several years ago, there was one bedroom in our home that was extremely cold in the winter and smoking hot in the summer. The winter chill used to cause havoc with my chronic pain. I couldn't even get warm once I was under the covers at night. But we just adapted. Kim and I would complain to one another, yet we'd continue living with things the way they had always been. The following year we actually moved out of the bedroom for the winter into the guest room. Fortunately, we didn't need to move furniture, but all our clothes and personal possessions made the annual migration with us. It was much warmer in the guest room, and we were quite toasty once we settled in. We didn't give a moment's thought about the upheaval. We just accepted it as a perfectly natural thing to do. It became our annual bedroom shift.

Because we had totally renovated our place over the years, each of our three bedrooms had become the master bedroom at some point in time. They were all similar in size, so the only real difference was where the rooms were located. Our favourite was the back bedroom because it looked out onto the private back garden. It's not as though I spent a great deal of time looking out of the window, but each time I opened the blinds in the morning, I would see the garden and think how lucky we were to have a nice home. It would make me smile and put a good start on my day. By the time we got to the spring and things were beginning to warm up, I was always pleased to move back to our summer bedroom.

About the third or possibly the fourth year into our migratory pattern, I decided one day to call an electrician to see if there was a problem with the baseboard heater because it didn't feel like it was producing much heat when I touched it. I know I had touched the heater many times before doing routine cleaning, so you would have thought I would have sprung into action long before now. Within 48 hours, the electrician had visited and repaired the unit. I happily paid the $75 and we had blissful heat. We were so pleased. We moved back into our favourite bedroom that very evening and things returned to normal. We never experienced the seasonal bedroom shift again. When we finished renovating our home later that year, we put in insulation. The freezing and overheating issues took care of themselves once and for all.

Why didn't I realize I could take action to fix the entire situation? Why didn't Kim? I would like to think that both of us are reasonably intelligent adults quite capable of phoning an electrician. In fact, an electrician had been to our house on several occasions for other matters during this time and we didn't even think about getting him to look at the issue. Had we just become so accepting of the status quo that we didn't even look for a solution? That just might be the problem right there. We have all heard the phrase, "Can't see the wood for the trees." We must have been deep in the forest, that's all that I can figure.

We all likely have come across similar situations in our own lives; a poor wifi signal in one room of the house, an electrical outlet in an inconvenient place or a cupboard under the stairs that remains pitch black. We know the situation exists, we merely haven't sprung into action to rectify the situation. Now, when something isn't working, I am much more decisive and take action—and it feels good. Even the things I choose to do nothing about, I accept that on some level it must be working for me or I would have done something about it by now.

We first have to recognize that a problem exists. Not all of the problems I have encountered have been completely my fault. When I really dig through it all—and I mean using full-on heavy-duty emotional excavating machinery—I often discover that in some way I played a part in the predicaments that I found myself in and need to own my contribution.

Things really began to change for me once I began a dialogue with my body. Somehow, I had managed to sail through life without paying the slightest notice to my body. Well, until it forced me to pay attention to a broken bone or some routine medical ailment. I was a fix-and-then-ignore type of girl. I would put the effort into my recovery, only to return to the same pattern. It happened time and again, so is it any wonder that I found myself in the clutches of medical science?

Are you like I was, the only one who didn't show up for "My Body: An Introduction Class"? Fortunately, you can sign up at any time and at any age. You are never too old to learn something new about yourself. We only stop learning because we choose to.

Before you say to yourself that it's too late to do anything … I lost 4,384 non-refundable days lying motionless on the couch before I drew that line in the sand and said enough was enough. Once I finally started getting to know my own body, it began to find a way to heal and even forgive me —even though I probably didn't deserve it. I finally made myself the priority that I should have been all along.

Your future isn't written yet. My 4,384 days are now history. I can't change a thing.

Reconstruct the life you had or the life you planned for. Those broken pieces do not need to be scooped up into the trash bin and discarded. Instead, take those same broken pieces and transform them into a beautiful mosaic.

The difference between try and triumph is the "UMPH." Put the "umph" into creating the life that you want.

Mission Control, We Have Achieved Lift-Off

Now that you are able to acknowledge that a problem exists, the focus then turns to what you choose to do about it. I personally would not have been able to take that first fragile step forward if I had dwelled totally on logistics and how long it would take to turn my health around. Not to mention if it was even possible.

It is vital to understand that I didn't have all of the answers tucked away neatly in a trunk when I ventured forth on my great adventure. Heck, I didn't even have all of the right questions. I was beaten down and broken, lost amid the chaos of my own making. You don't always get the opportunity to have everything laid out perfectly with all the safety nets strategically in place. Sometimes you have to settle for awkwardly imperfect and take that leap of faith anyway.

Once I drew my line in the sand, I stopped convincing myself of all of the reasons why this could never work. I started instead to think exclusively about how it could work, and how I was going to make it work.

I admit that it is frightening to try something new, but it was every bit as frightening to sit and do nothing.

I believe that obstacles are the gift of character. I heard a lot of no's before I found someone who said, "I think that I can help you." Even then, he didn't make me any promises.

If you haven't found the right person to help you yet, make a list of who you have seen or what things you have already tried and look at it with fresh eyes. I didn't see one neurological specialist, I saw three. Each of them saw things a little differently. They weren't wrong, they were taking different approaches. It's human nature to ask for a second opinion. It's one of the very first things we do even as a child. If I didn't like an answer I got from Mum, I would ask Dad.

"Mum, can I go and play outside in the garden?"

"No, dinner will be ready soon," or "No, go and do your homework."

I then go find Dad, who is oblivious to the conversation I just had with Mum.

"Dad, can I go and play outside in the garden?"

"Sure, just be careful, don't forget to put on a jacket, and don't leave the garden."

"OK, I won't." I skipped out of the room, snuck past Mum when she wasn't looking and there I was in the garden as happy as can be. When you are little, the favourite parent is always the one that gives you what you want.

I knew that at some point, Mum and Dad would realize what just happened and I would be told to come in, but until then I was quite happy to get away with it for as long as I could.

Always choose the answer that gives you the best result, whether it's your parents, or even a health-care professional, to an extent. If I needed surgery because a bone was broken, there is no point in asking them if they minded asking a colleague to see if they agreed with the diagnosis, there has to be some common sense.

When I was going from specialist to specialist, I often heard, "I don't know," or "I think it might be..." When that happened, I treated the potential diagnosis as though it was another gem for my mosaic. I was piecing together a roadmap for my recovery.

What if you get it all wrong? What if you make a mistake? How many hours has each of us pondered that very thought? As much as we all try to avoid mistakes, setbacks happen and failures occur. There are just too many variables to be considered in order to successfully avoid them all.

Before you beat yourself up, don't forget that there isn't a person alive who hasn't made a mistake. It is impossible not to make mistakes along the way. If it helps any, I find generally that I learn more from my failures than my successes. The successes are great, but we are living in a fantasy world if we think that they will continue forever. My failures caused me to dig deeper into myself, taught me to stand up, dust myself off, and find a way to battle on.

Once you have established your list of who you have already seen, build one of the things you haven't tried yet. Ask anyone whose opinion you value not what they would do in your situation, but rather can they think of anything that you might be overlooking? The reason that I don't ask people what would they do in my situation is simple: they aren't in my situation and never will be. That might sound harsh, but it is true.

By all means, make the most of the camaraderie of someone who is in a similar situation as yourself, just keep in mind that we each bring our own life experiences and wisdom to any situation. What works for one person doesn't always translate for someone else. Harley would be the first one to tell you that he can't always duplicate his successes. Why is that? Surely all he has to do is tell someone what they need to do, show them how it's done, mix in some cheerleading razzle-dazzle, and presto, his job is done, right? Oh, if it were only that simple.

For one thing, a person needs to be in the right mindset to benefit from the expertise offered. Harley could have simply hung out with me for an hour and got me moving, job done. Even with him in control, as smart a man as he is, that wouldn't mean that our success would be guaranteed.

I wanted success badly enough that I removed every single logistical and emotional roadblock that I encountered— whether the roadblock was a boulder or an avalanche. I planned my workout times in the beginning so that my medication would be at its most effective. I chose a smaller private gym because I knew that, if I didn't, I would find a reason not to go. I knew that if I stopped going it would be game over.

I changed how I prioritize my health. I rarely said to Harley that I am not coming. I don't bail because a friend has suggested meeting me for lunch. Instead, I try to find a way to do both. I just alter things slightly and might go for a later lunch or meet up somewhere closer to the gym once I am finished. I don't want to miss out unless I have to. It's funny how things evolve over time. Now my friends and family ask me, "When are you meeting Harley because I was thinking we should get together for lunch soon?" When my sister and I went away, we planned it so that we went right after my workout and came back home before my next one a few days later. My sister loves me and as long as we got away, she didn't mind working it around what I needed to do.

When I go on vacation, I try to arrange it so that I see Harley just before I go and then again as soon as I get back. I make the appointment for my return even before I leave town. When I come back, I usually take a few days to settle back into my usual rhythm. If I am not careful, that could go on for weeks without an action plan. With my workout booked in advance, I am back into the groove in no time.

With that in mind, chart your own course. If you find someone who you think could help, make a plan to meet up. If not in person then by a video chat or phone call.

Have a clear idea of where you want to see yourself, or how you want the meeting to go. I find that seeing any type of specialist can be intimidating. In those types of settings, I tend to forget some of the questions that I had been meaning to ask, even though I always ran the questions through my head before my arrival. This would happen often enough that I put any questions I had into my computer before I went, printed them out, and brought them along. I always listened to what the specialist wants to tell me first, before glancing at my questions. If there was any question that hadn't been touched on, I would ask them. This way I made sure that questions that had been niggling away at me got answered. Dr. Welsh got so used to seeing me, that he would automatically look for my list of questions.

There is a time and a place for the internet. I never used to look up anything medical unless my doctor specifically told me to read up about something and gave me the trusted website to go to. For one thing, to me, it was all just medical mumbo jumbo. It rarely made any sense, and it invariably always ends up causing death! I am trying to avoid that for as long as possible. I didn't want the weight of what I read playing around in my head. It messes with my mind. I needed to be positive and the stuff on the internet was certainly less than positive. There is also a lot of false information online, or there is a risk that I might be reading something totally outdated.

Everyone knows there are medical breakthroughs all the time. For me, I needed an individual diagnosis that was specific to me. The internet is just too broad. When it comes to medical information, I always return to my trusted source, my family doctor. He can understand the variables that affect me specifically. Dr. Welsh is fluent in medical mumbo jumbo, and he can put things into words that I can understand. It wasn't so much about me sticking my head in the sand, as it was a matter of keeping my mind clear and my thoughts positive.

If you are someone who finds it a challenge to take it all in and make sense of what you are being told, bring a good friend along to be your extra set of ears. Take it from someone who knows, when you are emotionally invested, things get twisted and what you thought you heard wasn't what was said at all.

Don't keep silent if you aren't getting what you need. It isn't easy to tell someone that you aren't happy with your progress. But in my experience, it is kinder to tell the person so that you might find a solution than it is to have them believe they are doing a good job but you just stop coming.

Like any good relationship, it involves both give and take. It's so easy to fall into the trap of believing that if you are paying for something it should be your way. Or if you are seeing a doctor they need to follow your instructions. If you are seeing any sort of professional, then give them the courtesy to do their job. Only step in as a last resort and do it respectfully. I had many years of doing things my way, and look at what a fine mess I had dug myself into. You want to find someone who works with you, not just for you. Harley knows how to get the most out of me, not because he is psychic, but because he pays attention. I've given him the tools and he uses them.

One final thing I want to recommend is, whenever possible, don't write something off without exploring the pros and cons first. If someone had told me to work out with a personal trainer right back at the very beginning, I would have thought that they were nuts and would have dismissed the idea immediately. Look what I would have missed.

Life Preservers

There are life preservers out there, even where you least expect them. A case in point: Harley was booked to give a talk about the benefit of exercise to a local support group of people who were dealing with various chronic pain issues and how best to manage them.

Because Harley was well-acquainted with my story, he invited me to come along. He talked about exercise as it pertains to pain management.

Then Harley spoke a little about what he does as a trainer and medical exercise specialist. The talk was then opened up for me to speak about my experiences: how bad I had gotten and how things had changed for me since trying exercise. I was a poster child for what was possible with the right help, commitment, and positive outlook.

During the intermission, Harley and I were both surrounded by people who were eager to know how we had achieved success. I know that when I was in agony, I would have loved to have had the opportunity to talk to someone who had made it safely to the other side.

We were there for about an hour and a half or so, and the people attending were asking quite a few questions. I could feel their anguish as some of them told a little about what they had been going through. It brought one of the participants to tears as she spoke of her turmoil.

These were my people. It wasn't all that long ago that I was searching for the exact same answers that they were. It didn't matter what the origin of their pain was. They didn't have to have neurological pain in order for me to be relevant. Be it physical or psychological pain, by definition alone, pain is universal. I believe it is the primary way the body has of letting us know that something, is wrong no matter where the source originates from.

At the end of it all, Harley generously offered to provide not one but several complimentary sessions to the group to get them started. That was a lovely gesture. It would be a way to show them first-hand what he could do to help them. In the gym setting, he would have the right equipment and could provide a more personalized approach. All they had to do was contact him to set up a time that would work for the majority of them.

Because this would be something new for them, it was ideal to keep them together. There would potentially be less anxiety among them and they could be each other's support going forward. I was on board with it as well and offered to be there to cheer them on. It wasn't a sales pitch. There were absolutely no strings attached. Harley had even gone to the trouble of speaking to the gym manager and making arrangements to get them free access to the gym. Of course, he wasn't charging anything for his services, so as far as I could see there was nothing for them to lose. We simply wanted to make a difference and get people thinking about physical movement as part of their solution.

If it were me, I would have jumped at the chance, if for no other reason than I might hit on something that would work. Everyone thanked us profusely for coming, and with that, we left. Not a single person took Harley up on the offer. It's everyone's choice to make, but I couldn't help but feel that if even one person had dared to come and try even once, Harley might have been able to help them, even if only in some small way.

Even now, I think about that day on occasion, wondering what became of those people. Did they find a way out, or were they deep in the thick of things? Where are they now? I felt sad for Harley's sake, it must have been disheartening. He has experienced successes with some of his clients and sees the people who could benefit from what he can do. He had thrown them a lifeline and they failed to grab it.

Your lifeline may come in an entirely different form. If you aren't on the lookout for it though, it may pass you by entirely. Life preservers don't always come in the form of the round tube aboard every commercial marine vessel. For me, it was in the form of a confident and fit young man with a clipboard. Keep your eyes open and be ready. When your lifeline comes, grab firmly with both hands and hold on tight. Your very life might be depending on it.

Survival Kit

I couldn't possibly begin to tell you every success and every heartache I have encountered along the way. What I have included here are just snapshots of moments that have left their mark. Good or bad, they have all woven themselves into my life's story. Collectively, they have given me strength, character, and the ability to keep my pilot light functioning, no matter what storm I face.

For those times when life gets hard, it's a great idea to have a well-equipped survival kit ready to grab and go when something happens. The first thing that always comes with me is my tenacity and spirit. They are the fuels of my inner pilot light. Whenever I feel physically and emotionally depleted, they provide my inspiration and strength. I avoid bringing along emotional baggage, as it just takes up room and doesn't contribute anything.

I have a few things that might appear silly to an outsider, but I need them. For example, I have a theme song: "Fight Song" by Rachel Platten. To me, it's my rock anthem. It tells the story of my journey perfectly. If I ever find myself down, I play it. If I am on the exercise bike when it comes on, I spin faster with less effort. That burst of energy only lasts for the length of the song, but the option is always there to hit repeat and keep pedaling. If the song comes on the car radio it automatically gets cranked up. That song makes me fierce. My inner warrior princess somehow shines. It even gives me the courage to keep soldiering on when I need to. It really has a powerful effect on me. What would your anthem be?

I did not get to my worst point in just a day, not even in a year. It just snuck up on me until it became too large to ignore. By the time I took notice, I was already in a deep dark hole that didn't have any visible exit signs. When you are deep in the trenches, it takes time to discover a way out.

Ah, the power of time. We all want what we want when we want it, but life isn't like that. We have to be patient. Looking for temporary, band-aid solutions won't work. I am years into my ongoing health recovery and I work on it every day, for the simple reason that I am worth it. Be ready to play the long game. If your plan has a solid foundation the rest of the recovery program builds from there.

Pack some good work clothes. If you want something, you have to be willing to work for it. Fight for it if need be by any means possible. Put on those work boots, grab your hard hat and sledgehammer, let's go! If you are anything like me you will find as in any restoration project it starts with the demolition phase.

This phase was filled with both apprehension and elation. It's unnerving to take that first swing of the sledgehammer, but once you have done, the swings keep on coming. It's a brilliant form of therapy. The years of frustration anger and resentment fade into nothing. Everything that you have hated about your existence is now a pile of rubble at your feet.

Here comes the fun part, the clean-up, and rebuild. When the slate is clean and you have a blank canvas to work with, the possibilities are limited only by your imagination.

I wanted my health back more than anything else I have ever wanted. It doesn't get given to you. I needed to put in work that only Harley and I knew had to be done.

The exercises that I used to do back at the beginning are easy for me now, they would be the warm-up exercises to my warm-up. I am not reliant on those earlier exercises anymore. They are a previous version of my Harley Knows Best list. My list is always evolving. My current list is every bit as challenging as those earlier ones were, it's the content that changes. There will always be work to be done.

Dare yourself to be unrecognizable. Sure, when we look in the mirror at ourselves, we see more grey hair, a new wrinkle, or perhaps an extra pound or two. When we don't recognize who we have become, that's a different thing entirely. The human that I was as a young child would not recognize me during my sedentary rock phase—just as the couch dweller wouldn't recognize who I have become now. I would like to think that the future me will be an even better version of who I am now. I know one thing for sure, I'm going to be younger.

Don't forget to bring along your supporting cast. Kim and Harley have both played starring roles in my life story. Even with star power like that, there were other roles that needed to be filled. It was friends and family who were the glue for my mosaic masterpiece. It's easy to feel alone when you are dealing with a chronic illness. Fortunately, I didn't get a chance to be lonely. The kindness of everyone was every bit as effective as any medication I could take.

I had calls from England almost every day. One cousin went so far as to specifically get a calling plan to Canada, even though mine was the only number ever called. Telephone calls were a brilliant distraction for me. It would give me a small view of the outside world. I would get lost in enjoying their company. The next thing you know an hour had flown by, that one gesture has stuck with me. Whenever I know someone is having a challenging time I always try and stay in touch, it's a small gesture of paying it forward.

About once a month my sister would take me out for the day. We usually had a nice lunch together somewhere and did whatever shopping needed to be done. If I required anything though any other time, I only had to text or call her and she would do whatever she could to help.

Those in my inner circle were the people who stuck with me. People like my friend Jennifer were life-savers. We met when we were teenagers at work and have been friends ever since. There was one Christmas day that we were both working until 9:00 p.m. I wasn't going to get a proper Christmas dinner, because I had to be at work before our family Christmas dinner would be ready, and it would be long gone by the time I got back home again. Jennifer invited me to come back to her place for dinner because her parents were waiting until she got home to eat. So there I was 9:30 at night on Christmas day sharing a holiday feast with her Mum, Dad, and younger sister. I never forgot that.

It will always be a special Christmas memory.

Jennifer enjoyed studying reiki, which is an Asian practice of healing with energy. When she wasn't working, she would come over from time to time and give me a reiki session to alleviate my pain and brighten my spirits. All the while we would have a nice visit catching up on what she and her husband had been doing for fun. We also would go for a pleasant car ride on occasion. Like Kim, she was very in tune with how many hours I was spending at home alone in the house.

I have been on both sides of the equation as a part-time caregiver for my aging parents and as someone in need of a caregiver myself. Honestly, neither role is easy. When my Mum was in palliative care, I stayed with her every chance that I could. There was one time though that I just needed to be somewhere else. My plan was to be as fast as I could, grab a quick bite to eat, and then return to my post.

When I returned, I found an off-duty care worker sitting beside the bed holding Mum's hand. I had tears running down my cheek. Mum was just lying there. It was only her pacemaker that was rhythmically keeping her alive. This angel of a person looked up at me and was almost apologetic for being there. She said that she had finished work and knew that Mum was alone. Her husband and children weren't going to be home until late, so she just thought she would keep my place with Mum until I got back.

Another friend from out of town was here visiting their own family on a flying visit. They knew things had taken a turn for the worse with Mum, but didn't know what care home she was in. They called around town to each care home until they found me. I got the biggest hug, had some more tears, and they drove off again. They must have been there for 15 minutes at the very most. That is unconditional friendship. They brought fuel for my fire. In the words of Paul McCartney and the late John Lennon, I get by with a little help from my friends.

Your survival kit will be different than mine, contents might vary but whatever you personally need will be in there the moment you reach for it. What are you waiting for? Make a list and then head out on your scavenger hunt. You will be glad that you did should anything unexpected happen.

Give and Take

I'm like most people, I don't have an excess of money. I consider myself blessed to be able to afford the cost of a personal trainer and gym fees. It comes down to priorities when it comes to spending the money that is left over once the essential food and shelter costs are paid for. I make my health a priority. Without health, it doesn't matter how much money I have in the bank: I have nothing. I happily go without eating out whenever I feel like it or having 200 channels to watch on the television. Besides, that many channels would lead to too much sitting.

Where I live, there is a program at the local recreation facility which is open to any low-income individual or family. Anyone meeting the income thresholds can apply to have 52 drop-in sessions per year for free plus you can get a reduction on any programs that you want to do four times a year.

Whether it's for your emotional or physical well-being, you can't beat free. No matter where you live, enquire if there are any similar programs that are available and if you qualify. What have you got to lose?

I personally think that our health-care system should cover the cost of providing everyone with their very own Harley if they want one. Once we graduate from high school it's up to us to try and remain active. It's unfathomable to me that the government believes that twelve years of physical education classes in our youth are enough to last a lifetime. When you consider that people are living up to 100 years of age and even beyond, that's up to a good 80 years that we are left to our own devices. No wonder our medical system is in such shambles. Don't let your fingers be the only thing you exercise playing video games or texting.

If you can't afford a personal trainer, all is not lost. Start perhaps by finding a friend who works out and ask if they can show you a few things to get you started. You could also see if your local trainer is willing to work with two of you together. The fact that it would mean that he or she can't spend all of their time on one person can be outweighed by sharing the experience with a friend.

One thing that surprised me about joining the gym was how willing people are to share what they know. They are a fabulous group of cheerleaders.

They know what it takes to create new abilities and likely have a few tips or tricks to share that they have picked up along the way.

Our local Taoist Tai Chi society offers a health recovery program as well. If you are having difficulty physically moving right now, then let your brain get a workout. Check for groups that might be able to help. Ask a friend if they know anything that can help. If they are friends like mine, they will be delighted that you asked. It's what everyone who loves you has been waiting for.

While we are on the subject of people helping people, it is a two-way street. Why not look into the countless volunteer opportunities that are available in your neighbourhood, if you haven't already. It's a great incentive to move off of the couch. It got me out mixing with the world, rather than watching the world as if I was in an alternate universe. It restored my sense of purpose. I felt appreciated and it took me out of myself. I have had such a sense of personal satisfaction from volunteering. It not only helps the charity, but it also helps me. There is a multitude of charities to choose from no matter where you live. Just pick one that touches your heart like Autism, Parkinson's, or your local cancer centre perhaps. Where I live there is a local website full of volunteer opportunities, that are just waiting and hoping for people to volunteer. There is something to fit everyone's interests and abilities.

If structured volunteering isn't your thing, might I suggest offering to pick up groceries for someone when you are doing your weekly shopping. If a neighbour lives alone and finds it hard to make a meal, next time you make a little too much, put the extra on a plate and surprise them. I know Kim used to do income taxes at the senior centre each tax season, even though accountants are customarily smoking busy at that time of year. He met so many people who were worried about getting their taxes done, they didn't know where to start. It was a big deal to them and for Kim it was straightforward. Kim got the satisfaction of helping and the senior got much-needed peace of mind.

If you are unable to get out of the house, you can still make a difference. Try FaceTiming or Skyping someone. It can feel like a mini-visit and could easily brighten your day, just as much as it will for the person you contact. The possibilities are only limited by your own imagination.

Normal You Say! What is That?

I have a real aversion to the words, "It's your new normal." For me, it's like the sound of nails running down a chalkboard. It just sends me over the edge. Even the support class that I went to in order to learn how to deal with pain implied just get used to it, it is your new normal. I couldn't buy into that notion at all. I was years into hell at this point and couldn't find a way out. This can never be normal. I won't allow it. To call it normal to me was surrender.

This was years before the Covid-19 pandemic, which hijacked the phrase "the new normal" and gave it a far more serious connotation. Those words now imply that the world as we knew it at the beginning of 2020 no longer exists. It is now up to each individual no matter where they are in the world to create a reality that they can learn to become comfortable with.

The only masks that I remember having in the house prior to Covid were found in our first aid kit. Now one is with me whenever I leave home.

Personally, I find the whole thing more mentally exhausting than anything else. We are all continuously weighing the risk, assessing the pros and cons of any activity that is outside of our own homes.

I, like millions of people, had never heard of Wuhan, China. Pandemics seemed a world away from my quiet little life. Things can and do change overnight. You only need to look at the onslaught of Covid-19 as proof of that. When I began this book, things were as they had always been. Life was ordinary, perhaps even pleasantly boring. In a matter of weeks, the entire world changed. From the way we conduct ourselves, how we interact with people, how we do business, it has all become unrecognizable.

This is, without doubt, the clearest example that we are ever likely to experience of life's ability to change in a heartbeat. It was global. Billions of people are affected. If this doesn't tell us to grab life with both hands and seize the day, I don't know that we are ever likely to experience what will. You can't always wait until tomorrow to take action. The journey forward can't begin until you take the first step, no matter the size of the step or how tentative it may be, your journey will have begun. Even during global chaos, we have the power to create the world that we want for ourselves.

If Mother Nature has her way, the global impact of Covid-19 will have changed everything. From the way we think to what we do, and to what is important, both for the planet and we humans that inhabit it. We will all be a little different, and that is not in itself a bad thing. We can be part of that change.

Now the phrase "the new normal" has had a resurgence. We have no choice but to find a way to adapt. We have to find a way to become comfortable with our new reality. Covid-19 changed us all in one way or another.

We might be adjusting out of necessity, but what if we changed things because of choice. Imagine how powerful that would be! That's fuel for everyone's fire.

In the early days, my gym closed, seeing Harley wasn't possible. For the first two or three weeks, I pretended that it was a holiday from the gym. It was a pleasant change of pace. I kept in touch with Harley mostly by email, but I didn't really have too much to report. A pandemic was the perfect excuse not to concentrate on my health. I wasn't ignoring it, it just wasn't front and centre in my thoughts.

Up until this point, I hadn't thought about what I needed to do in order to limit the damage that being sedentary was doing. I just wanted a break. Other people were doing it and I felt I should be among them. Surely, I could take it easy on myself without any consequence for a few weeks. I should be back to the gym in no time.

I did do some exercise, but it wasn't purpose-driven. I wasn't pushing myself to the edge of my physical capabilities like Harley would have been doing. Even before a worldwide pandemic, I couldn't make myself work out with the same intensity that Harley gets out of me.

I was just a few short weeks into self-isolation when it happened. Suddenly out of nowhere, that familiar surge of pain occupied my body. I had been having the pains on and off for years, accepting that fact as just something that was going to happen from time to time. I was disappointed to feel it, but not entirely surprised by its appearance.

The pain was worse than it had been in quite some time. It was a bunch of jolts all in quick succession. Oh my God, what if this is only the beginning? Had it been waiting for a moment when I took my eyes off of my health to take up permanent residency again? The thought of it was alarming. Is an exercise vacation worth it? Had I gambled with my health and lost? It took a Herculean effort on my part to stop my mind from racing that day. I couldn't see Harley even if I had wanted to. Holy crap, what now?

Fortunately, even though I couldn't see him, Harley hadn't shut himself off. I had all his contact details, I just needed to reach out and let him know what was happening. I didn't want to tell him. I reasoned that it was my mess to dig myself out of, but how could I do that? My body was missing Harley and the gym, and it was letting me know it. I took a deep breath gathered my courage and began composing the e-mail. Thankfully he replied quickly.

There was no, "I told you so," instead he simply reminded me that I needed to commit to doing my workouts from home. It might not be the same as the gym, but I could prevent or at least control the pain outbursts, I just had to simply do the moves. It is far from easy to make yourself do something that you don't feel like doing. I can relate to the people who lament that they have tried and failed to achieve their goals for the exact same reason, it feels like too much work.

Harley asked me to list all of the exercise equipment that I had at home, then he adapted a few things so that I could do the majority of the exercises that I was doing at the gym from home. It was surprising just how much equipment I had gathered or the everyday household things I could use to get the job done. Fill a couple of used milk jugs with water and I would have a set of weights, or even lifting those family-size containers of laundry detergent can up the intensity of the workout. I just needed to be creative. It wasn't costing anything as we already had these things. Home workout equipment became scarce very early on, so alternatives had to be found. Even though exercise equipment was in my basement ready to use, it didn't mean that my mindset would follow suit. I was obviously doing some exercise but not enough. After a few e-mails and a pep talk phone call from Harley, I realized there was no other option but to make my home workout the priority even when there was no one else making me do it. I needed to be enough.

I am sharing this with you in hopes that it demonstrates that setbacks can happen when you don't expect them. As long as you keep your survival kit at the ready though, hopefully, what would previously have caused a derailment, is now nothing more than an annoying hiccup.

Harley told me that he wanted to hear from me daily about what exercises I have been doing and how things were going. In true Harley fashion, he told me that I could have one day off a week. At first, I could only think that this was crazy. How the hell could I keep motivated by myself within a pandemic?

Pain can either fuel the passion for success or it can crush you. Mentally the pandemic zapped my strength initially, but I wasn't going to allow the years of hard work that I have done to end up being for nothing. I scaled back a little and began to rebuild. I had told friends that I was emailing Harley every day with updates, and more than one person suggested that I just tell him what he expected to hear, just fudge the results. That sounded tempting, but I knew at some point he would eventually see me and know in an instant that I had been lying to him. It turned out that Harley's request for daily updates ended up being a very good suggestion on his part.

Let's just say that it worked for me. I managed to get everything back on track. I have no way of knowing if he actually read the emails each day, he might have just skimmed them for all that I know, just in case I asked something important, but that doesn't even matter. It kept me accountable. While everyone else was sending delicious-looking photos of what they had been baking, I bonded with my Harley Knows Best List as though my life depended on it.

As the pandemic continued to drag on longer than anyone ever imagined or wanted, I bucked the trend and actually lost both weight and inches. It was five months of not seeing Harley at all before the local medical authority lifted the restriction and allowed in-person workouts to resume at the gym. My greatest fear of meeting up with Harley was that my body wouldn't know what hit it when I saw him and was put through my program for the first time. Part of me was excited to give him his job back. I never wanted to be my own personal trainer, that's for sure. I have always appreciated Harley and now that I know how much more difficult it is going it alone. His job training me is guaranteed for many years to come.

When I think about all the work it takes to stay on top of my health issues, it could easily put someone off from trying it themselves. I can't blame anyone for wanting to run. What I like to remind myself on those occasions is simply this: being unhealthy is a hell of a lot of work.

Navigating a downward health spiral can easily be as difficult as climbing one of the world's highest mountain peaks. It, too, takes a mental and physical toll on you just like any mountaineering adventure.

Whether it's some sort of new normal or not, why settle? Why would anyone settle for something that they don't want? You can work hard to do nothing or you can work hard to claim the life you want rather than the one that you have. Sometimes it's all about compromise, I get that, I will compromise on something like what side of the bed I am going to sleep on or what TV program we are going to watch. I won't compromise when it comes to regaining my health. Even if global pandemics get in the way and I stumble a little. I am worth the effort. We are all worth the effort.

Parting Thoughts

There is no one perfect thing that has made it possible to be where I am at this moment. I wonder sometimes about how things might have turned out differently if even any one of the choices that I have made would have been different. If I had gone to a different gym, or perhaps I hadn't waited for Harley to get back from vacation that day. If I had chosen to do nothing, would I be alive today?

If it was simply a matter of making up your mind and just doing something, you would accomplish a great deal more than any of us do. What is the difference then between a pleasant thought and taking action? Why is it that the thought you have had running around in the back of your mind for weeks or even years, suddenly has more weight? It takes on a sense of urgency.

Suddenly that one little thought has a spotlight shining brightly upon it. If you are wondering where the spotlight came from, that is your pilot light. Even when you introduce total darkness the light still beams brightly like a lighthouse in a storm. It is there to guide you safely home.

That beacon of light and hope is always with you. It stands at the ready should it be called upon and jumps into action when you truly need it.

It is that often-forgotten sparkle that we had in our youth when the world was full of wonder and ours for the taking. Before the weight of financial pressures and adult responsibilities cast its shadow. It's achieving the impossible simply because we never got the memo that said it couldn't be done.

Our inner spark can get buried under the chaos of our lives, but it is there, we haven't lost it. It's likely that we have simply forgotten that we had it in the first place. It is our misplaced treasure. It was tucked away in a corner somewhere because we didn't think at the time that we were going to need it.

Now that you know my story, I'm hoping that you have seen how important your inner spark is and what a difference it makes. It is integral to well-being.

The work continues. I am keeping my promise to be better to myself. Each and every day I diligently work to maintain my health, gain new physical abilities, and then maintain them by integrating them into my everyday life. I probably won't ever say that I am well enough to walk away from the gym and turn my back on all the successes that becoming mobile has given me. It has become a lifestyle shift that is still evolving. If I were to stop now, it worries me that it wouldn't take long before my life would once again become unrecognizable and I am not willing to find out how long that would be. Why would I let myself slide backward when I am wiser now?

There are pain patterns still bubbling under the surface and it wouldn't surprise me if these patterns are always going to be with me in the shadows, in one form or another. Neurologically whatever has been causing the brain to initiate these pain surges has never been properly resolved.

You won't always get a definitive answer to a complex medical condition no matter how much you might want one. For me, that remains the case. So instead of giving up, I had to look beyond standard medical care and think outside the box. Over time, I have been able to adapt to a hybrid of fitness and old-school medicine.

I remind myself that there are things you have no control over; however, you always have control over how you want to deal with it. I am now firmly the one in control.

The game-changer, without a doubt, was calling in an expert and then listening to what he had to say. I am fortunate in my case to have chosen the right man for the job. There will be more challenges, those are unavoidable, but through all of this, I have developed so many more ways to live my life on my own terms.

I am willing to go wherever this journey takes me. Things really began to change for me once I began a dialogue with my body. It took so long for my body to get me to pay attention. Now that it has, it remains my central focus. I need to keep myself strong and healthy so that I can now help others that might find themselves back where I was that night at the hotel drawing a line in the sand saying that enough is enough. To them I say, "I hear you."

There are so many achievements yet to be celebrated. I want to see what I am capable of. Through all of this, I have come to learn that sometimes, travelling along a difficult path may be the only option to get to where you need to be. It is just that simple.

I have Harley in my corner, and hope I will for years to come. Together we are on the warpath, ever ready to battle the mighty pain demon. If you want to know more about the work that Harley does, check out his website for updates: **Preston Wellbeing, soma-x.com**. The hope is that he will write his own book about the science of fitness. His will likely become the much-needed missing instruction manual for the human body. He is after all a technician, a true movement mechanic.

As you continue on in your own journey may your pilot light always shine brightly.

In Gratitude

Kim and Harley, for graciously allowing me to tell our mutual stories. The fact that you didn't ask me to change a single word is a true testament to your belief in me.

My family, for being there through it all with your love and support. I couldn't have done it without you. I love you all.

Mum Skelly, for teaching me from a young age that "everything's meant." It has changed the way I see things and has gotten me through the very darkest of days... but most of all thank you for creating our Kim.

Penelope Ball, for believing in me, inspiring me to put pen to paper and creating the lovely cover art.

Marianne, for showing me how to turn my life story into this book, and for generously agreeing to be the voice of the audio version.

My Cheerleading Crew, I heard your cheers loud and clear, you kept me going and I think you are amazing.

Simone, you coaxed the words out of me. You challenged me to revisit some difficult memories for the benefit of finding the missing chapters that I had so conveniently buried. You have brought my words to life.

Sue, you are always there for me through thick and thin. For knowing all of my flaws and loving me anyway.

Carol and John, you have done more for me than I could ever put into words. I don't think you can ever totally know how much it has all meant to me.

The Maundrell Clan, for all the time we have shared together and the lovely memories it has given me. In the middle of a bad night, I knew that you were someone I could call if I needed to. It is the only upside to distance and time zones.

The Rogers Clan, for all the special memories that we have created over the years. May there be many more. We have been through a lot together. Through it all, you were there with handkerchiefs ready or flags waving. I am so thankful to have you as dear friends.

Jenny and Jeff, for reiki visits, the laughter, and allowing me to escape my world and simply enjoy sharing your world for a bit.

Dr. Welsh, you know who you are. For all the times you have gone to bat for me, for translating medical mumbo jumbo, and for looking after my physical well-being so very well.

Kelly A, you are one of a kind. Your lightness of spirit is effervescent. You make my world brighter.

The Singh Family, you have opened your home and your heart to both of us. You are such special people.

Treasured friends, your generosity of spirit, your wonderful unexpected meals, the visits, and your words of inspiration have enriched our lives beyond measure.

My gym family, you make me feel like I belong. You encourage me to always aim high and inspire me every day to be the best that I can be. I love the camaraderie and our shared spirit of genuine friendship.

I am bound to forget someone, and if that someone is you, please accept my humble apology. On a journey that has been years in the making and still continues, it would be a book all on its own to list all of you. Know though that although you weren't mentioned specifically, you did make a difference. Whether it was the smile that lifted my spirits when I needed it or the knock on the door to check if everything was alright. I thank you so very much.